HYPERACTIVE CHILD

HYPERACTIVE CHILD

Belinda Barnes
& Irene Colquhoun

Thorsons
An Imprint of HarperCollinsPublishers

Thorsons
An Imprint of HarperCollins*Publishers*
77–85 Fulham Palace Road
Hammersmith, London W6 8JB

1160 Battery Street,
San Francisco, California 94111–1213
First Published by Thorsons 1984
This edition published 1997

1 3 5 7 9 10 8 6 4 2

A catalogue record for this book
is available from the British Library

ISBN 0 7225 3531 7

Printed in Great Britain by
Caledonian International Book Manufacturing Ltd, Glasgow

ACKNOWLEDGEMENTS

The authors owe a great debt of gratitude to Sally Bunday, who founded the Hyperactive Children's Support Group (HACSG) and who is still actively involved in running the group.

PUBLISHER'S NOTE

While there is no risk of side-effects in following the self-help approaches suggested in this book, it is very important that parents consult their family doctor to ensure that no fundamental medical problems are being overlooked.

This book is presented as informational and educational material. It is not intended as medical advice, and in no way excludes the necessity for a diagnosis from a health professional. Although care has been taken to ensure the accuracy of the information presented, the authors and publisher cannot assume responsibility for the validity of all of the material or the consequences of its use.

Throughout this book the authors use the pronoun 'he' when referring to a child. This is not to overlook the parents of girls affected by hyperactivity, but merely to make unnecessary the use of the more cumbersome he/she.

CONTENTS

FOREWORD

There is a right and a duty for all children who live in our developed, western world to receive an adequate education which should, in due course, allow them to take their place in adult society.

Mothers and fathers who have developed, through necessity, many stratagems to entertain and coerce their hyperactive child to curb his excessive behaviour, must be aware of the difficulties experienced by the caring Reception Class teacher when confronted by her new pupil.

There are perhaps fifteen children in the Reception Class, all in need of attention, but the hyperactive child needs much more than his allotted time. He finds it difficult to concentrate, and fidgeting is second nature. His writing is poor because of lack of motor control, he is quite likely to be clumsy in the classroom and inadequate at games. At this point of low self-esteem the child can become very disruptive, often trying the patience of his hard-pressed teachers and classmates to the limit.

Teachers are becoming increasingly aware that the number of learning disabled children is growing at an alarming rate. No longer can we just pass these children off as 'naughty', 'badly brought up' or 'stupid', as has so often been done in the past. Here is a case where constructive help to alleviate the situation is desperately needed.

The HACSG is spreading a philosophy of hope to all parents and teachers who come into contact with the group. First there is the relief of knowing that you are not alone with your problems, and secondly there is a wealth of practical knowledge, amassed by years of experience in dealing with hyper-active children, to draw on.

Hyperactive children who are put on a carefully planned diet of simple foods almost always improve on an all-round basis. There seems no predictable rule as to the form this improvement takes. For some the effects are dramatic and immediate, for others slower and more painstaking. As general health improves, so fewer school days are lost for minor ailments. Parents are rewarded with a calmer child and the teacher is encouraged by a child who can now sit still long enough for teaching and learning to take place. Slowly, lessons are learned and manual techniques mastered. With the improvements come moments of success and break-through which are immensely rewarding for the young person who has known mainly failure to date. Following each success comes the motivation to achieve even more, and the process of education begins to take its due course towards the production of a well-rounded, integrated adult.

Having taught hyperactive children for some years it seems to me only right that all concerned with the future of these children should have the opportunity to read this book, to understand what may have gone wrong with the finely balanced machinery of the child's system and hopefully set all children back on a better path towards health and well-being for the future.

Valerie A. Ehlers
Specialist Remedial Teacher

INTRODUCTION

In centuries past children's health was threatened mainly by infectious diseases, ignorance of basic hygiene, bad sanitation, impure water, and poor nutrition. Epidemics of cholera carried children off in their thousands, and other waterborne diseases, such as diphtheria and enteric fever, raged in the cities. On a less stupendous scale scarlet fever, measles and whooping cough accounted for many childhood deaths. In fact at one point things were so serious that an Act of Parliament was passed in 1875 decreeing that no child under the age of five years old could be insured for more than £6.

Help came when harmful bacteria were identified and methods of immunizing against them were developed. Infectious diseases are now largely a thing of the past – hence the closing of the special fever hospitals.

What has happened in recent years, however, is that a large number of other adverse factors have entered the environment. These have led to conditions such as hyperactivity, dyslexia and other learning disabilities, and a great increase in chronic illnesses such as asthma, eczema, epilepsy and digestive disorders. Perhaps the most difficult of these conditions in the family context is hyperactivity.

THE HYPERACTIVE CHILD

Unless one has lived with a hyperactive child it is easy to assume that 'hyperactive' means a rather energetic and boisterous child. This is far from the truth. Almost from the day the child is born there are problems, and, if it is a first child, the parents have no idea what could be wrong and all too often blame themselves for being inexperienced.

The utter misery and chaos caused by such a child severely disrupts and damages family life. Many marriages break up, and we suspect that some cases may end in 'baby battering'.

The Hyperactive Children's Support group (HACSG), a registered charity, has for over 20 years responded to thousands of requests from distraught parents, desperate for help.

The hyperactive child lives in a constant state of over-stimulation or, some would have it, under-inhibition. For reasons we will later investigate, his central nervous system is in a permanent state of 'go'. The hyperactive child is constantly moving – running, walking, climbing and bouncing about. He is quite unable to sit still and attempts to make him do so will result in hysterical outbursts. His activity will continue even when he is overtired and overwrought to the pitch of tears and tantrums. Even when he is exhausted he finds it hard to sleep. When he does drop off he tends to sleep lightly and restlessly, and wake early. He may often wake in the night, crying and screaming for reasons he cannot explain.

Any form of stimulation may encourage feverish excitement which will escalate into hysterical behaviour and often end in screaming and crying. He is very easily stimulated and very hard to calm down. Instructions are ignored, he cannot concentrate on a task for more than a second, and attempts to pressurize him will lead to outbursts of anger and frustration.

The parents know that their child has a severe problem that is causing him and them endless distress, but the casual observer will probably dismiss him as a 'spoilt brat', and place the blame on him or his parents.

So far we have described the severely hyperactive child. As with all physical conditions, there are degrees of severity, from the severely afflicted child to the mildly affected. There is no magical 'cut-off' point beyond which a child is hyperactive and before which he is not hyperactive.

Symptoms of hyperactivity

Not all hyperactive children/adults will suffer every symptom listed at one and the same time – they may vary in number and intensity. From puberty onwards or earlier some children seem to improve, but from our limited knowledge of adult hyperactives there are certainly quite a number of residual problems such as insomnia, abnormal thirst and lack of ability to concentrate.

From the Hyperactive Children's Support Group surveys it appears that many hyperactive children come from families with a history of 'allergies', hay fever, eczema, asthma and, in a large number of cases, mothers with migraine.

Hyperactive children often seem to suffer from 'colic' as small babies, sometimes with eczema, asthma, ear, nose and throat problems, rhinitis (catarrh), tummy problems, etc. This is possibly because their immune system is not fully developed. (Hyperactive children are often immature in many aspects in relation to their chronological age.)

One of the symptoms which we have found in a high percentage of hyperactive children (male and female) is an *abnormal thirst*.

GROUP 1: BEHAVIOURAL DISORDERS
1. Constant motion
   May walk on toes

Runs not walks
Rocks or jiggles legs
Cot rocking, head banging

2. Excitable, impulsive behaviour
   Unpredictable behaviour
   Panics easily
   Cries easily and often
   Whining, clinging behaviour
   Intolerance of failure and frustration
   Demands must be met immediately
   Diminished ability to experience pleasure

3. Poor sleeping habits
   Nightmares
   Has difficulty getting to sleep
   Easy to awaken
   Cries out in sleep
   Fears sleep
   Often abnormally thirsty

4. Short attention span
   Inability to concentrate
   Flits from one object to another

5. Compulsive aggression
   Disruption at home and at school
   Compulsive touching of everything and everyone
   Disturbs other children
   Molests pets
   Destructive (toys, household articles, structural components)

6. Cannot be diverted from action, even if life-threatening
   Punishment of no avail (leads to frustration or tantrum)

7. Mutilation
   Scratching, biting
   Picking, tearing skin

8. *In older children*
   Lying
   Abusive language
   Stealing
   Arson (occasionally)
   Withdrawal
   Delinquency
   Fighting (conflict with peers)

GROUP 2: MUSCLE INVOLVEMENT
1. *Gross muscle*
   Clumsy
   Trips when walking
   Collides with objects
   Inability to play sport, cycle, swim

2. *Fine muscle*
   Poor eye/hand co-ordination
   Difficulty with buttoning, tying, fastening, writing,
       drawing (some children can draw beautifully but are
       still clumsy, i.e., they do not have all symptoms)
   Speech difficulties – stuttering, stammering, poor pro-
       nunciation
   Reading – dyslexia

GROUP 3: CLINICAL PATTERN OF COGNITIVE AND
PERCEPTUAL DISTURBANCE
1. Auditory/memory deficits
2. Visual/memory deficits
3. Poor comprehension
4. Disturbance in optical orientation (up and down, left
   and right)

5. Difficulty in reasoning (simple maths problems, meaning of words)

WHAT CAUSES HYPERACTIVITY?

Many factors recently introduced into the environment appear to be contributory causes to the epidemic of hyperactivity.

Heavy metal contamination

Heavy metals, for example lead, are antagonistic to essential minerals in the body such as zinc, manganese and chromium which activate enzyme systems. From conception, the child is at risk from heavy metal contamination. For example, the lead content of the air we breathe has risen sharply, due particularly to the lead content of petrol and also to the increase of car ownership in Britain.

Both lead and excess copper in a mother's body can affect the nervous system of a child before birth, as may cadmium from cigarette smoking, or aluminium from saucepans, food cooked in aluminium foil containers or drinks from aluminium cans.

Factory agriculture

Factory farming has led to an alarming assortment of chemical imbalances in our food. Oversimplistic soil-boosting fertilizers, containing mainly nitrogen, phosphorous and potassium, encourage the rapid growth of plants which alters the trace mineral content. The plants grow at an unnatural rate and so do not take up as much of such trace minerals as zinc, manganese, chromium, selenium and magnesium as they would normally do. This means there is a lower level of these minerals in the foods, even normal natural foods.

Non-degradable insecticides have been designed to destroy choline in the insect's body, thus preventing it from taking up manganese (which is necessary for the function of the nervous system) and thus eventually killing it. Such insecticides may have a similar cumulative effect on the human body. Manganese deficiency is frequently found in hyperactive children and children with allergies. Herbicides kill the macrobacteria in the top soil, inhibiting uptake. Macrobacteria facilitate the uptake of minerals. Wheat may be induced to produce more grain per head by hormone manipulation. Then a hormone inhibitor is introduced to restrict growth of the stem, as the heavy grain will otherwise blow down in rough weather.

Antibiotics in milk and meat come from the routine doses given to cattle to prevent infectious disease. Antibiotics destroy intestinal flora (bacteria necessary for digestion) in the human gut, thus interfering with the normal breakdown and assimilation of food.

In addition, extra hormones are given to promote rapid weight gain in animals. Chemicals may be sprayed on fruit to prevent it ripening too soon; sometimes the fruit is later dyed to look riper than it is.

All these chemicals, and those added by the food manufacturers, add up to a formidable bombardment of the immature gut and central nervous system.

Alcohol

The consumption of alcohol has risen in this country over the last twenty or thirty years, especially among young women. It is well documented that the use of alcohol in pregnancy may result in retardation with hyperactivity in the baby. The precise amount of alcohol, if any, that can be taken during pregnancy *without risk* is not yet known.

Smoking

Smoking in young women – and men – has increased, as has the use of so-called 'recreational' drugs. All are known to have a deleterious effect on sperm and ova development, and on the central nervous system and skull formation in the developing foetus.

Artificial additives

In recent years many scientific studies worldwide have been carried out with regard to the effects of artificial colourings, flavourings and other preservatives and additives, such as sweeteners. Products such as monosodium glutamate are added to food not to enhance it in any way, but to artificially stimulate the taste buds of the consumer. Many of these additives may be eaten together in the course of a day. The effect of such combinations shows that these additives can affect *behaviour*, *health* and *learning* to the detriment of thousands of infants and children[1] ... and, to a certain extent, adults.

The UK allow the *most* 'E' number additives in foods – approximately 300. However, with EU harmonization we understand that the additive lists of every country (in the EU) are being combined (harmonized) to produce a 'super list' of 411.

Some additives do not have 'E' numbers. However, flavourings, the biggest group of additives and the major category of *non-E-numbered additives*, do not have to be listed separately by name on labels even though in the UK alone there are 3,700 in use.[2]

Drugs

It is well known that such drugs as 'tranquillizers' have the very reverse effect on a hyperactive child. What may not be so well known is that in many major cities the tap water will have been 'purified' and recycled many times. The residues of these drugs may be present in the drinking water from the urine of people who have been using them. Added to this we are told to flush unwanted medicines down the lavatory. When the water is then recycled for further use, it may not be entirely safe.

All of these pollutants, and no doubt many more we are not yet aware of, combine to have a devastating effect on the immature central nervous system of today's child.

Nutritional Deficiencies

At the same time as an ever increasing number of chemicals are being added to our daily diet, and drinking water, research shows that essential nutrients are being extracted from basic foodstuffs during processing.

For example, from what used to be known as 'the staff of life' (the ubiquitious loaf of white bread), there has been removed: 87 per cent of the chromium, 91 per cent of the manganese, 81 per cent of the iron, 70 per cent of the cobalt, between 70 per cent and 90 per cent of the copper, 83 per cent of the zinc, 50 per cent of molybdenum and 83 per cent of the magnesium that would be found in a whole wheat loaf. In addition, much of the B complex vitamins and vitamin E are removed. Of thiamin, vitamin B_1, 77 per cent is removed, 80 per cent of the riboflavin is removed, 81 per cent of the niacin, 71 per cent of the pyridoxine, 50 per cent of the pantothenic acid, 67 per cent of the folic acid and 86 per cent of the vitamin E. All of these nutrients are essential for the digestion of wheat: as we eat the white bread, they are leached from our body's reserves. All are also essential for maintaining normal central nervous system and brain functioning.

THE EFFECTS OF LIVING WITH
A HYPERACTIVE CHILD

Unchecked and untreated, environmental poisons and dietary deficiencies can play such havoc with the nervous system of a tiny child that these children can, from babyhood, be exhibiting atypical behaviour which in an older person would be recognized as a severe degree of mental illness. To live all day with someone who may be unable to keep still, unable to sleep, unable to respond to affection, who is subject to uncontrollable tantrums, who may constantly expose themselves and others to danger, who is unable to learn even simple tasks, and who does not respond to the spoken word, is something of an emotional marathon!

All parents (especially mothers) of hyperactive children are under an almost intolerable degree of stress which is seldom understood by the outsider. In many cases it may drive the mother to seek help from tranquillizers for herself, but in some mothers tranquillizers release inhibitions in her stressed nervous system, so that she may batter the child.[3] The HACSG therefore recommend very strongly that mothers under stress avoid these drugs, which often worsen rather than improve the whole situation.

THE HYPERACTIVE CHILDREN'S
SUPPORT GROUP (HACSG)

The Hyperactive Children's Support Group was founded in 1977 by Mrs Sally Bunday and her mother Mrs Irene

Colquhoun. It was the direct result of Sally's experiences with her own hyperactive son, her frustration at not being able to find understanding and help from the medical profession, and her feeling that not enough was being done for these children and their parents. (See Appendix 1.)

The aims of the group are to:

1. help and support hyperactive children and their parents (not financially);

2. encourage the formation of local groups or contacts where parents may get together for mutual support and understanding;

3. urge the medical profession, health and education authorities to take more interest in the day-to-day problems of hyperactive children and adolescents;

4. promote urgent research into causes of hyperactivity; whether it be linked to chemical food additives, nutritional deficiencies, food allergies and/or environmental pollution, and all forms of stress;

5. press for early and proper diagnosis of hyperactivity, possible treatments and management, and to disseminate information to all interested parties.

Why is a self-help group needed?

This is an important question. If such a condition as hyperactivity exists, why is it not recognized by the medical profession and subjected to scientific investigation? And why is help not available through the accepted channels? In our experience it is for the following reasons.

Recent changes in the amounts of chemical pollutants and poisons which enter our bodies, and the sharp reduction in intake of the nutrients needed to maintain growth, development and health, have led to a bewildering spectrum of effects on the human body. As the brain, central nervous system and endocrine system are part of the body, many of these changes manifest as severe problems with mental development and behaviour. Just as the more serious effects of physical disease are commonly seen in the very young or the very old, so we are finding the more disastrous effects of this manipulation showing in the very young as hyperactivity, learning difficulties, allergic syndromes or chronic illness. (Just as with the very old, senility and confused thought are becoming an increasing problem.)

The parents of the hyperactive child are therefore facing problems of which neither they, their parents, nor their GPs have had much previous experience. So there is virtually no one to whom they can turn for advice.

Most GPs have had no training in nutritional and/or environmental hazards and their subsequent repercussions. For the most part they have no understanding of nutritional therapies, allergies, mineral metabolism, or the effects of cranial anomalies or fluorescent lighting on the central nervous system. They have no choice therefore but to prescribe drugs or to recommend psychoanalysis.

In the past, drugs[4] have proved neither effective nor completely free from harmful side-effects.

With psychoanalysis the situation is even more confused. A common result of misapplied and misunderstood psychoanalytic theories is that parents seeking help with a problem child are often subjected to indifference, implied blame and rudeness. Indeed, it appears that research into biochemical causes of hyperactivity and other mental illnesses has been severely inhibited and hampered by these attitudes.

This, briefly, is why lay organizations have had to step into the gap. We are hoping these attitudes will change as medical practitioners, and other professionals who look after these children, become more aware of the genetic, biochemical and metabolic/environmental causes of hyperactivity. HACSG has been a pioneer in this dietary/nutritional approach/biochemical, with good success.

In the meantime the HACSG continues to gather information. In this book we have brought together all that we know so far about methods of treatment which many hundreds of parents have tried and found to be invaluable.

The added bonus of the approaches we suggest is that they very often bring improved health to the whole family.

Notes

1. This has been documented by Dr Ben Feingold of California. Dr Feingold has hypothesized that familiar and beneficial minerals such as zinc and manganese might be used by the body to 'coat' foreign substances to ensure them a safe passage through the kidneys or liver; HACSG research tables.

2. *Food Additives: A Shopper's Guide* (Channel 4 and BBC Support Services).

3. It was recorded in a letter in the *British Medical Journal* (1 February 1975, p.26) that 92 per cent of mothers who battered their babies were on tranquillizers. The letter was in response to an article which appeared in the issue of 18 January 1975 on the side-effects of commonly used tranquillizers.

4. A long list of drugs was noted from questionnaires returned to HACSG by parents of hyperactive children. These had been prescribed by the doctor. After dietary intervention, many of the children were able to discontinue their medication. However, in the past two to three years, many

hyperactive children in the UK have been prescribed strong *psychostimulant drugs*, which research shows give short-term relief. In a review in the US where these drugs have been in use for many years, extensive research has shown that these drugs have no significant beneficial long-term effects, either in social adjustment or academic achievement. There are some minor and some significant side-effects. Furthermore, according to the manufacturer's data sheet, these drugs should not be prescribed for children under six years of age, as the research into safety and efficacy has not been carried out.

CHAPTER 1

THE SELF-HELP PROGRAMME

The HACSG has studied a great deal of background work on hyperactivity, learning difficulties and disturbed mental development, and the therapies developed to offset these problems.[1] From what we know at present we believe that parents should look for and correct the following factors in the hyperactive child.

1. Nutritional deficiencies, particularly vitamins of the B complex, A, C, D, and E, calcium, magnesium, manganese, zinc, chromium, selenium, cobalt and **essential fatty acids**
These nutrients are to be found abundantly in fresh wholefoods, especially in diary products, fish, meat, poultry, salads and fruits eaten raw, wholegrains, nuts, pulses and sprouted seeds. They are *noticeably deficient* from many convenience foods. (See Chapter 2 for diet suggestions.)

Of the first seventy mothers who replied to a questionnaire sent out by the HACSG, sixty-eight had found significant improvement in the child from following this régime alone. Sleeping problems improved and hyperactivity was very significantly reduced. For some children (particularly those who live in a comparatively unpolluted area) following a diet of fresh wholefoods entirely free from artificial additives, and eliminating certain obvious factors from the environment (e.g. aluminium saucepans), is sufficient for the child to improve. Other children need further investigation.

2. Sensitivities to food allergens and to pollutants, and coeliac disease
The withdrawal of certain foods and/or external factors which affect the child adversely can also bring an improvement. (We will discuss this further in Chapter 3.)

3. Heavy metal toxicities and trace mineral deficiencies
Many children suffering from hyperactivity have been found to have a high body level of toxic metals. Often this is lead or aluminium, more rarely it is mercury, cadmium and/or over-high copper. High levels can be detected by hair analysis and then reduced by a cleansing programme and by supplementation of vitamin C and specific trace minerals. The same analysis will reveal trace mineral deficiencies – these can be replenished by supplementation. (Further details are given in Chapter 4.)

4. Facial defects and skull deformities, including the high raised palate
Some hyperactive children have long, narrow 'pinched'-looking faces, with pointed chins, overcrowded teeth, and low-set protruding ears. The top teeth may be pushed forward and the chin may recede.[2]

Many hyperactive children (possibly because they were short of essential nutrients in the womb) may also have somewhat poorly formed asymmetrical skulls and high raised palates. This type of aberrant skull formation may inhibit the flow of blood and cerebro-spinal fluid to the brain cells and thus impair the supply of oxygen, blood sugar and other nutrients. A high raised palate may put pressure on the base of the brain.

A controlled study by Mr Colin Dove, of the British School of Osteopathy, was carried out in collaboration with a consultant psychiatrist, with a large number of retarded children in an NHS hospital. Mr Dove and the psychiatrist in charge found that a programme of cranial osteopathy helped children with high raised palates, and/or malformed skulls.

In recent years some osteopaths and chiropracters have found that disturbances within the flexible infant head are responsible for faulty postural development, and can influence bodily functioning especially through subtle effects on the brain.

It is thought that after the use of forceps during delivery, or other unusual trauma, such as a difficult, prolonged or sudden birth, the separate platelets of the skull might not be able to move freely. Babies who have had a traumatic birth experience frequently manifest hyperactive tendencies.

A very large number of HA children suffer from serious ear infections, and it has been found that osteopathic treatment can help and reduce the need for surgery.

Cranial osteopathy practised by a properly qualified osteopath has been found to be very helpful for some HA children. Help from a qualified chiropractor may also be helpful (see Useful Addresses). Such treatment can lower a high-raised palate and reduce pressure on the base of the brain.

5. *Adverse reaction to fluorescent lighting*

The work of John Ott[3] suggests that fluorescent lights, and in some cases the rays from the television tube, may have an adverse effect on the central nervous system of hyperactive children. This needs further investigation but the possibility is one more thing to be borne in mind by parents who are trying to help their child. If he seems to react unfavourably to fluorescent lighting, try to rely on daylight or other forms of artificial light as much as possible, and avoid exposing him to a fluorescent bulb for long periods of time.

Television viewing should also be kept within limits. During the summer months the child should be encouraged to play outside as much as possible. (As research progresses the HACSG hopes to have more information on this particular subject.)

The self-help programme

Presdisposing factors
Poor nutrition, severe stress, allergy or illness in pregnancy are very important factors when it comes to hyperactivity, as are stress or trauma during birth. Nutrient deficiency in the womb can lead to failure of the baby's brain to develop. A noted authority has written, 'whereas it was initially believed that early malnutrition led to permanent behavioural scars, current data suggests that changes are reversible ... That nutritional interventions may be effective means to alter brain chemistry and thus, behaviour, is more than a tentative conclusion.' Restoring nutrient status, while cleansing toxic metals, chemicals and other pollutants from the child's system, and providing a basically healthy lifestyle, will in most cases largely reverse the damage. In other words, more often than not the child's body will use the added nutrients to 'catch up' in areas where development has been lagging.

Basic strategy
Foods: The most important step is to get the child onto a nutritional wholefood diet, as laid out in Chapter 2. This diet consists of fresh wholefoods, and excludes all artificial flavourings, colourings, etc. However, the child may not take well to a natural diet if he has been used to a lot of sugary foods. Many will be very picky, some disinclined to eat, and some downright hostile to the idea of coming to the table at all!

Initial supplements: In order to get anywhere, therefore, the vital thing is to improve the child's appetite. Zinc (which is an important trace element needed for appetite) and B complex vitamins are very important in this battle. We would suggest, for the first two weeks, adding a few zinc drops and liquid B vitamins to drinks that he is willing to take. Good response has been found using Ziman Drops containing zinc, manganese and vitamin B_6 in correct amounts: Two drops per day per stone in bodyweight, plus BioCare liquid multivitamins (a comprehensive vitamin supplement for children) at 4 drops per day per stone in bodyweight. (See Useful Addresses for details of BioCare.)

If this is accepted, additional Essential Fatty Acids (EFAs) in the form of Evening Primrose Oil drops (1 drop per stone in weight) plus a pinch of vitamin C powder once per day may be stirred into juice. The choice of juice is quite crucial for hyperactive children, as they are often affected by 'salicylates' (naturally occurring in some fruits). Pear, lemon or pineapple juice should disguise the taste of the drops quite well.

Hyperactive children often suffer from abnormal thirst, but this should decrease once they are on a better diet plus the supplements, especially the EFAs.

After a couple of weeks on the drops, the child's appetite should have improved quite markedly, and the time is right to start gradually to cut out the foods containing white flour, sugar and colourings, and replace these with more nutritious foods. Discuss foods with your child, if he is old enough. Tell him some of the things he likes will have to go, as they are bad for him and making him ill, but you will search together to find nice things to replace them.

Check the list of good foods in the following chapter, as well as the menu suggestions. These are just suggestions, to try and give you lots of ideas – not rules to be followed slavishly! Read them through with your child, and try and inspire him. Even at two-and-a-half, children can get quite interested.

Tell them the good foods will help them to grow strong, to have nice white teeth, to be clever and (if this applies yet!) to be a success at school. (Yes, they will, have faith!)

It may be a good idea with younger children who are poor chewers to purée the food for a bit. Poor chewing is a sign of under-development due to lack of zinc. If, because of this, they eat very little, this compounds the problem. As they get good nourishment, normal development will be accelerated and puréeing will become less necessary, but some may need to have their meat shredded up for a long time.

Buy organic foods whenever you can. Many major supermarkets are getting more organic foods all the time. The more we all buy it, the cheaper it will get. It is free of pesticides and has much greater trace mineral content. (See Useful Addresses for organic suppliers.)

Drinking water: Filter all drinking and cooking water. Jug filters will remove a significant amount of lead, cadmium, aluminium, copper, pesticides, nitrates, oestrogens and excess chlorine. It is also possible to purchase 'whole-house filters'. However, this is a major expense and may only be felt justified if your household water is found to be heavily contaminated and/or if your child has eczema and reacts very badly to bathwater.

Food additives: Harmful food colourings have some of the worst effects on the hyperactive child. Foresight has brought out a small handbook called *Find Out*. This details the adverse effects, supplying colour-coding for: 'Harmful/ Conflicting Reports' and 'No Known Adverse Effects'. The supermarkets are now much more aware of the colourings issue, and most at least try to avoid the hazardous ones in 'own brands'. We are not 'danger-free' however, and this may remain the case while there is huge money to be made from junk foods – and from the medicaments they make necessary!

Fresh air: Along with fresh foods and clean water, try to see that your child gets plenty of fresh air. Any windows that do not overlook a road with heavy traffic should be kept open a bit all the time. Always be sure that your child sleeps with an open, though guarded, bedroom window. It may be necessary to get vertical bars put over the window – hyperactive children may climb up horizontal bars! Sleep small wrigglers in vests, sleeping suits and long jerseys. Try and take him for a good walk (run!) in a field or park well away from traffic every day if possible, so he has time for both exercising and breathing comparatively clean air. All this will help his appetite.

Smoking: It is important that both parents stop smoking, as the effects of smoke can be very profound on the hyperactive child. It can act as an appetite-depressant (which will put a huge block on his recovery) and also as a cause of asthma, and epilepsy. Smoke is not good for any child, but for the hyperactive/allergic child it is disastrous.

Gas: If you have gas appliances in the house, get these checked out. Some hyperactive children are especially sensitive to even very tiny amounts of leaking gas. Try to minimize any escape when you light gas rings, etc. Have the lighted match ready and apply it at once.

Lighting: Fluorescent lighting has been found to exacerbate hyperactivity. Limit exposure whenever this is possible. Some schools have fluorescent lights in the classrooms. Discuss whether this is affecting your child with his teacher, and what can be done about it.

Urinary Tract Infections: Some associated health problems crop up frequently. A number of these children have urinary tract infections. In some cases these may stem from infections caught in the birth canal during the birth, such as chlamydia, ureaplasmas and mycoplasmas. If the child is small, irritable and tearful, and has difficulty keeping dry day or night over the age of two-and-a-half years, or if the urine has a strong odour, or gives him a rash, then it is as well to check this out by taking a sample to your GP for examination.

High raised palate: Ask your dentist whether your child has a high raised palate, or compare his palate with that of his friends. An asymmetrical skull, a very laid back forehead or a markedly receding chin are all quite easy to spot. If in any doubt, get this checked out with a cranial osteopath. A few sessions of gentle massage will be helpful in restoring the balance of the skull – and will often improve your child's prevailing mood!

The supplements as described, and these few simple aids to restoring normality, may be all that is needed with many children. However, there are some who need more detailed help, and for these we would advise as follows:

- Check for food allergies with a qualified practitioner – either an allergist or a trained nutritionist. (See Chapter 3.)

- Have a hair analysis and a detailed programme of supplements tailor-made for your child (details of this approach are given on page 63).

Notes

1. Much of the practical research was done by Dr Ben Feingold and Dr Elizabeth Lodge Rees of California, Dr Abram Hoffer and Dr Glen Green of Canada, Dr U. Blackwood of Ohio, and the late Dr Weston Price of California. Helpful dietary advice has been found in the papers of the McCarrison Society, The Henry Doubleday Association and The Soil Association.

    We have also been helped in our work by the books of Dr Richard Mackarness, Dr Carl Pfeiffer and Dr Henry Schroeder, and many others writing on allergy and diet.

    Animal studies that we have found helpful have included the work of Dr Bert Vallee of Harvard University Medical School, Drs Oberleas and Caldwell of Wayne State University, Michigan, and Dr Lucille Hurley of the University of California.

The above scientific papers can be obtained from the Foresight Library. Write to Mrs Jill Clarke, 8 Duchess Close, Strood, Rochester, Kent.

2. These features have been clearly described and photographed by Dr Weston Price in *Nutrition and Physical Degeneration*, his book about the effects of a refined diet on children's bone structure. He ascribes ill-formed bone structure to the low level of calcium and fat soluble vitamins in our Western diet. His research was limited as techniques for measuring trace minerals were not available to him in the 1930s.

3. See John Ott's *Health and Light* New York: Pocket Books.

CHAPTER 2

NUTRITION

In this chapter we want first to take a general look at food and then discuss in detail vitamins and minerals. The rest of the chapter sets out general principles for planning meals, followed by detailed menu suggestions and recipes.

We have found that many hundreds of hyperactive children respond very favourably to a varied wholefood diet entirely free from chemical additives. The recommended diet eliminates excess sugar (extra sugar means extra hyperactivity). Food is only sweetened when absolutely necessary and then with raw Barbados sugar or Muscavado sugar, honey or molasses, used very sparingly. It is a good idea to vary the diet as much as possible and *not rely too heavily on wheat and milk products, as these are very common allergens in the hyperactive child.* (See also Chapter 3.)

For simplicity we have divided food into four main groups – cereals, vegetables and fruit, meat, dairy products – and will look at 'good foods' and 'foods to be avoided' within each category.

ORGANIC FOODS

Many members of the HACSG have found that organically grown food has greatly enhanced their child's improvement.

CEREALS

Good Foods

Wholewheat bread, i.e., bread containing 100 per cent of the grain. Some bread is merely refined flour coloured with gravy browning. Check labels or with your baker, and don't accept anything less than wholegrain!

Some hyperactive/allergic children cannot tolerate wholewheat bread or wholewheat breakfast cereals (may cause aggressiveness in some children). Please be watchful of *all* wholewheat products.

If at all possible buy *organically-grown* cereal foods, as wheat for instance is often sprayed a number of times during the growing process.

Wholewheat rolls, scones, cakes.

Wholewheat cereals, e.g. *Shredded Wheat, Shreddies, Puffed Wheat*, and all natural muesli cereals (beware of those with added sugar).

Porridge – made from pinhead oatmeal, millet, wholewheat meal, pot barley, maize meal.

Wholegrain crispbreads, e.g. *Ryvita, Vitawheat*.

Wholewheat biscuits, oatcakes, etc. (Biscuits can be made at home using wholewheat flour or oats with raw sugar or molasses, see page 38.)

Flour – whole maize (polenta), yellow and green split pea, potato, rice, sago, tapioca or soy. Almost any white flour recipe can be adapted to suit these ingredients.

Pastry – 'brown' pastry is difficult to handle; compromise with ⅔ wholewheat to ⅓ refined flour. (81–85 per cent stone-ground flours are also available.)

Tapioca, sago, wholewheat semolina, wholewheat pasta.

Foods to be avoided

White flour and all white flour products, e.g. cakes, biscuits, pastries, cake mixes, pudding mixes.

VEGETABLES

Hyperactive children are often seriously affected by salicylates (chemical cousins of aspirin) and have to avoid certain fruits/vegetables/herbs. These are marked with a double asterisk ** in the lists that follow.

Good foods

Raw vegetables and salads[1]
All fresh vegetables can safely be eaten raw except potatoes and some pulses. It is a good idea for a child to have a raw

salad every day. Salads can contain any of the following, whole, chopped or grated: lettuce, endive, chicory, white or red cabbage, cress, cauliflower, radishes, tomato**, cucumber**, celery, onions, carrots, button mushrooms, Chinese leaves, watercress, small peas, sweet peppers**, and all sprouted seeds like alfalfa and mung beans.

For flavour add all types of fruit**, dried fruit**, nuts, seeds, and fresh herbs.

Salad dressing can be made with sunflower seed oil, honey and a few drops of cider**, or tarragon vinegar. Home-made mayonnaise, yoghurt or soured cream can also be used.

Avocado pears are particularly rich in vitamin E, and all leaf vegetables are good sources of linoleic acid, an important essential fatty acid. Both these nutrients assist the take-up of trace minerals and are very important to the hyperactive child.

Cooking Vegetables
Where cooking is necessary, the following guidelines will help preserve vitamins and minerals.

1. Vegetables should be picked as short a time as possible before the meal (if home-grown) and then washed quickly and cooked immediately.
2. Where possible vegetables should always be scrubbed with a soft brush rather than peeled or scraped.
3. Cook vegetables in as little water as possible.
4. Use the cooking water for gravy, soups, or stews, as it contains a lot of goodness.
5. Invest in a 'steamer'. All vegetables taste better if they are steamed rather than boiled.
6. Keep cut surfaces to a minimum, so that vitamins/minerals are not leached out.

Potatoes are best baked or steamed. Other vegetables can be stir-fried in a little sunflower seed oil (or similar) and the oil served with the vegetables.

Pieces of bean sprouts, celery, carrot, nuts, sunflower seeds, fresh or dried fruit**, etc, can be used instead of sweets. Vegetable and natural fruit juices** can be used in place of squashes.

FRUITS

A number of hyperactive children react badly to the salicylate-containing fruits. (Salicylates are chemical 'cousins' of aspirin and can build up in the body.) Omit all fruits listed below. After a good response to the diet (say eight weeks) introduce them *one at a time* and if there is no poor response, add them gradually, introducing them occasionally and not too much at any one time.

> *Salicylate-containing fruits*** include: almonds, apples, apricots, peaches, plums, prunes, oranges, tomatoes, tangerines, cucumber, blackberries, strawberries, raspberries, gooseberries, cherries, currants, grapes, raisins.

Good foods

All other fruits (including bananas, melon, pineapple), dried, fresh, home-frozen or stewed.

Home-bottled fruit (bottled in water only).

Home-pressed juices.

Cooking fruit
Fruit is best stewed in a glass dish in the oven or in an enamel saucepan. If necessary use a little raw sugar, honey or molasses.

Foods to be avoided

Fruits tinned in heavy syrup, which has a lot of extra sugar, may have lead from the seams of the tins, and in some cases artificial colouring.

Raw potatoes or potatoes that have turned green with frost – these contain nitrite which is a poison.

Tinned vegetables, which will have lost all vestige of vitamin C.

Commercially-frozen peas and beans, which may have been treated with EDTA before freezing, which removes trace minerals.

Vegetables cooked the day before and reheated – the vitamin C content will be nil.

MEAT

Good foods

Fresh meat, bacon, ham (*ask your butcher if these contain nitrates and other artificial preservatives – if they do, avoid them*), liver, heart, kidney, tongues, game, most poultry, deep-sea fish, and fish roes.

Fresh sausages free from preservatives – a local butcher may supply these, but check that they are free of preservatives and artificial colouring.

Pâté – made at home from fish, lamb's liver, or free-range poultry liver.

Meat from organic farms is best but may be hard to find although it is getting easier all the time. Enquire locally, see the Useful Addresses section at the end of this book or apply to the Foresight Association for information. (The Wholefood Shop, 24 Paddington Street, London W1 supplies it.)[2]

Meat should be bought as fresh as possible; venison, rabbit, game bird, pigeon and quail and all sea foods are the best meats nowadays as the animals have not been intensively farmed. Sheep are less intensively farmed than beef, pig products and chicken. The latter may have been subjected to artificial fattening and/or extra copper in feed processes and hormones to stimulate weight gain, etc. They should, therefore, be used more sparingly.

Cooking meat
Meat is best spit-roasted, grilled or stewed with vegetables and pulses, preferably in bone stock. The stock will then contain many of the minerals and should not be thrown away, but can be eaten with a spoon or used later for soup. Bone broth made from simmering joint bones, poultry carcasses, etc. is valuable for calcium and makes delicious gravy or soup.

Foods to be avoided

Stale meat and meat fried in stale fat.

Twice-cooked meat.

Tinned meats which contain sodium nitrate.
Commercial pâtés, packet bacon, ham, sausages and pies which contain preservatives and sometimes monosodium glutamate. (Some tinned sauces for meat contain monosodium glutamate and preservatives.)

Ready-cooked frozen meats and fish coated with artificially coloured breadcrumbs, batter, etc.

Capons and intensively-reared turkeys who may have been given extra hormones to promote unnaturally fast weight gain.

DAIRY PRODUCTS

Many children react badly to cow's milk and its products these days, possibly because the promotion of bottle-feeding has lead to earlier and earlier weaning on to a sugar and cow's milk formula with resulting adverse reactions. Some babies are still fed with cow's milk in the first few days of life in hospital. This section is for the more fortunate to whom cow's milk is a good friend. Egg white may also cause allergic reaction – in some cases eczema and asthma.

Good foods

Free-range eggs – they have more flavour and harder shells. The membrane surrounding the yolk does not break so easily when you try to fry or separate them. This all indicates a hen has been allowed to pick and peck all day long at will and has taken in a better diet with more trace mineral content than that of the pathetic prisoner in the battery. Fresh eggs keep for a couple of weeks, so it is worth making a journey to get them.

Organic milk yoghurts – most supermarkets now stock them.

Cheese, *except* those which contain preservatives or colouring (as some processed cheeses do).

Butter, *except* those containing artificial colourants.

Goat's milk, cheese and yoghurt. The fat in goat's milk is much nearer to human milk fats than the fat in cow's milk. The milk can be served as milkshakes made with bananas, honey, cashew nut butter, etc., or permitted pulped fruit**.

Ice-cream – Many supermarkets/health shops do stock suitable products, but check labels.

Fruit soufflés, syllabubs, fruit** 'snows' made with whipped white of egg.

There are, of course, no end to egg dishes and the changes can be rung with eggs from ducks, geese and guinea fowl – all of which are less likely to be intensively farmed. Quail eggs, in season, are delicious and research suggests that they may be useful in combating certain types of allergy.

Foods to be avoided

Tinned evaporated milk from tins with lead seams.

Dried milks, as exposure to light and/or drying destroys lysine, arachidonic acid and some of the B complex vitamins, all of which are important to the hyperactive child.

VITAMINS

Each vitamin has a different role to play in nourishing the body. Vitamins are divided into two types, the fat-soluble ones – A, D, E and K – and the water-soluble ones – C and the many Bs. The fat-soluble vitamins can be stored in the body in quite large amounts. The water-soluble vitamins are most vulnerable. They cannot be stored to any great extent and therefore need to be replenished daily.

Vitamin A

Role: good for the eyes, the internal membranes. It is needed for normal growth and contributes to a healthy skin, hair and nails.

Found in animal tissues which contain pre-formed vitamins, dairy produce (milk, butter, cheese), egg yolk, liver, kidneys, fatty fish and fish-liver oils. Man can also synthesize this vitamin from carotene which is found in leafy vegetables such as chard, kale, spinach, broccoli, string beans, carrots, tomatoes, marrow, red peppers, apricots, peaches and sweet potato.

Destroyed by strong light, heat, long, slow cooking, dehydration. Wilted vegetables lose a high percentage of carotene. Liquid paraffin prevents its absorption and should be avoided.

Vitamin B group

At least five of this group are needed to break down glucose and produce energy. They are needed for the metabolism of carbohydrates (sugars and starches), fat and proteins and to maintain the central nervous system. Deficiency in adults can cause depression, inability to concentrate, insomnia, 'mania' and other forms of mental breakdown. *The B complex vitamins are particularly vital to the hyperactive child as one of their main functions is to regulate the central nervous system.*

Separate vitamins improve muscle tone, regulate digestion, guard against constipation, utilize sugar, militate against allergy and perform many other vital functions in the body. One vitamin, nicotinamide, alone performs forty-two separate functions! Lack of the B vitamins can lead to complete physical and mental breakdown, but they are all removed from commonly used modern foodstuffs by the refining process.

B_1 *thiamine*
Found in brewer's yeast, wheat germ, whole grains, whole cereals, nuts, peanut butter (though please note that peanut allergy can produce severe, even fatal, reactions), dried peas, beans, soya beans, lentils, pork, ham, kidney, heart, liver and eggs.
Destroyed by cooking and storage in a warm place. It is quickly lost in an alkaline medium.

B_2 *riboflavin*
Found in brewer's yeast, milk, butter, yoghurt, cheese, eggs, whole grains, wheat germ, soya beans, peas, lentils, cooked leafy vegetables and lean meat and liver.
Destroyed by light.

B_3 nicotinamide
Found in brewer's yeast, wheat germ, whole grains, nuts, peanuts (avoid if allergic), eggs, green vegetables, fish, lean meats, liver, kidney, potato.

B_5 pantothenic acid
Folic acid and biotin are needed for absorption.
Found in brewer's yeast, wheat germ, whole grains, bran, green vegetables, liver, kidney and heart.

B_6 pyridoxine
Found in brewer's yeast, wheat germ, bran, molasses, liver, heart, kidney, peanuts (avoid if allergic) and mushrooms and just under the skin of potatoes (peeling potatoes may totally remove it).

B_{12} cynocobalamin
Found in milk, cheese, eggs, fish, most lean meats, liver and kidney. Vegetarians are more likely to be lacking in this vitamin. Vegans must use supplements.

Folic acid
Found in milk, nuts, all green vegetables, brewer's yeast, liver, kidneys.
Destroyed by cooking and food processing.

Inositol
Found in brewer's yeast, wheat germ, whole grains, oatmeal, corn, molasses and liver.

Choline
Needs pantothenate (B_5) for absorption.
Found in wheat germ, egg yolk, brewer's yeast, green vegetables, legumes, lean meat, brains, liver, kidneys.
Destroyed by an alkaline medium.

Biotin
Found in brewer's yeast, milk, eggs, mushrooms, liver and kidneys.

In practice most B vitamins are found together, and eating whole grain foods, with possibly the addition of brewer's yeast, either in gravies, soups and stews in powdered form, or as tablets, should ensure a steady supply. Eggs and green vegetables are particularly rich sources, as is toasted wheat germ, which can be sprinkled on cereals and salads.

Antibiotic therapy affects the supply of these vitamins because the drugs kill the normal intestinal bacteria which help us to digest food. One of the reasons why hyperactive children so often react to milk may be that the level of antibiotics in the milk could be interfering with the absorption of vitamin B. A deficiency of several of the B group of vitamins leads to skin problems. This *may* account for the fact that when children with eczema come off milk many of them improve.

Vitamin C

Role: necessary for the functioning of collagen – a substance which holds the cells together. It is very important therefore for healthy tissues, blood vessels, bones, teeth and gums. It also helps combat fatigue, counteract infections, remove toxins from the body. It also helps the absorption of iron.
Found in citrus fruits**, guavas, peppers**, pimentos, rosehips**, tomatoes**, cabbage, fresh strawberries**, salad greens, Brussels sprouts, broccoli, apples**, bananas, lettuce, potatoes, peas, blackcurrants**, sweet corn, melon and grapes**.
Destroyed by storing, soaking and boiling. Frozen foods lose vitamin C after they have thawed for an hour. Cooking once and later re-heating destroys it completely.

Vitamin D

Role: assists the uptake of magnesium and calcium, so contributing to the growth and solidity of bones and teeth.
Found in dairy produce – butter, cream, milk, fatty fish, eggs, fish-liver oils. *If* the natural oils of the body are on the skin (i.e., not following bathing), vitamin D can be made by the body in conjunction with sunlight. Cow's milk has about half the vitamin D content of human milk.
Destroyed by liquid paraffin which prevents its absorption.

Vitamin E

Role: necessary for maintaining suppleness and toughness of all skins, linings of the body, and muscle tone.
Found in wheat germ oil, whole wheat, milk, egg yolk, unrefined vegetable oils, green vegetables, especially lettuce and avocado pears.
Destroyed by rancidity in fats.

Vitamin K

Role: essential for clotting of the blood.
Found in cauliflower, spinach, kale, alfalfa, soya bean oil, and pig's liver.

Bioflavonoids

Role: thought to assist in maintaining blood vessel walls.
Found in citrus fruits**, grapes**, blackcurrants**, and rosehips**.

MINERALS

The body needs minerals for numerous functions. Hair analysis of hyperactive children has shown that they have a short supply of most minerals – in particular magnesium, zinc, manganese and chromium. When the lacking vitamins and minerals are adequately supplemented, many hyperactive children improve enormously.

Calcium

Adequate intake is important from birth to death.
Role: essential for bone growth and calcification of the infant cartilages and teeth; for heart muscle function, for contraction of all muscles, for the substance holding body cells together, and correct function of some cell membranes.
Found in milk and cheese. Where these are not tolerated, calcium orotate or Dolomite tablets should be taken daily. Also in apples, bananas, oranges, green vegetables, eggs, potatoes and carrots, bone broth or jelly, whole grain products, fatty fish – herrings, sardines, salmon.
Deficiency can cause pain in the joints, brittle bones and poor teeth.

Elderly arthritic adults who have eaten white bread (which has chalk instead of calcium) for decades, improve spontaneously over about a year when they change to whole cereals. Chalk may not be an acceptable substitute to all bodies!

Magnesium

Role: helps transmit nerve impulses to muscles. Is necessary for the growth and repair of body cells. It has been found to help children to become calmer and more responsive to the spoken word. It is a vital component in numerous biochemical reactions.

Found in nuts, soya beans, green vegetables, whole grains. Vegetable water from cooking should be kept and consumed.

Deficiencies can inhibit brain development, increase vulnerability to infections and can cause muscle twitches, cramps, tremor and emotional irritability.

Iron

Role: essential for the oxygen-carrying constituent of blood.

Found in brewer's yeast, wheat germ, whole grains, egg yolks, fish, red meat, liver, raisins and all dried fruit**, green vegetables.

Vitamin C is necessary for complete uptake of iron in food. For children who are not salicylate-sensitive, apples are helpful (they contain malic acid which helps iron absorption) and/or raisins soaked for twelve hours in lemon juice.

Iron cooking pans may contribute trace amounts.

Copper

Role: necessary for the efficient absorption of iron from food and for brain development and function. Since the invention of copper water-pipes, deficiency is less frequent. Needed in minute quantities and generally sufficient is absorbed from food or water. However, often found to be at very low levels in hair of autistic and retarded children. This may sometimes be due to prolonged use of medication to control epilepsy, and is worthy of further investigation.

Manganese

Role: essential for growth and skeletal development. Carries oxygen to the nucleus of the cell and is essential for correct brain function. This includes thought, memory and concentration. Frequently found to be *very low* in the hair of hyperactive children and epileptics. Both conditions respond to supplementation (see p. 27). Choline, pantothenic acid, folic acid, biotin, vitamin B_6, essential fatty acids, and vitamin E are required for absorption/usage. Cantassium make a supplement, *Manganese Plus* to combine these nutrients in one preparation.

Found in nuts, whole grains, dried fruits, green vegetables, seeds, bran, brown rice, oats, buckwheat, onions, strawberries**, bananas, apples**, pineapples, green beans, liver, snails(!), poultry and seafoods.

Chromium

Role: needed for insulin to utilize glucose.

Found in brewer's yeast, whole wheat, liver, beef, beets, beet sugar, molasses and mushrooms.

Deficiencies found in 'reactive hypoglycaemia' and diabetes.

Zinc

Role: needed for cell multiplication, i.e., mental and physical development. Found to be especially important in pregnancy, puberty, teething and when fighting infection. Essential for healthy growth, skin, wound healing, hair growth, and acuity of taste and smell.

Found in all raw vegetables, especially peas and carrots, green vegetables, nuts, a small quantity in all fruit, liver, lean meat, chicken, whole grains, wheat buds, bran, oatmeal, eggs, milk, North Sea herrings and oysters.

Selenium

Role: essential for the skin and the pancreas. Important in the prevention of cancer.
Found in brewer's yeast, garlic, liver, eggs, brown rice, whole-wheat bread.

SUPPLEMENTS

Junamac is a supplement which can be given to children who need help to make up vitamin and mineral deficiencies more quickly. It is available from health food stores without a prescription.

For young children the tablets can be crushed and mixed in with food.

Junamac formula

Vitamin A	200iu	Folic acid	4mcg
Vitamin D	25iu	PABA	15mg
Vitamin E	30iu	Choline	60mg
Ascorbic Acid		Inositol	50mg
(vitamin C)	50mg	Biotin	2mcg
Vitamin B	2mg	Zinc	1.5mg
Nicotinamide	30mg	Manganese	3mg
Pantothenic acid	8.2mg	Chromium	2.9mg
B_6	5mg	Calcium	39mg
B_{12}	2mcg	Magnesium	8.67mg
		Phosphorus	13.86mg

Manganese Plus formula

Calcium phosphate (mineral, trace)	Potato starch
	Calcium pantothenate
Soya lecithin 80mg	15mg
Evening primrose oil	Vegetable fatty acid (trace)
66mg	B_6 3mg
Vitamin E 66iu	Natural vegetable gum
Manganese orotate 50mg	Biotin 5mcg
(supplying 6.5mg of	Folic acid 10mcg
manganese)	

Essential Fatty Acids

The brain and central nervous system are formed very largely of certain types of fat. These fats are found in abundance in human breast-milk, but are much less readily available from the feeding formula that is often given as a substitute.

Essential fatty acids cannot be made by the body and must be acquired through food. The polyunsaturate of overwhelming importance in the human diet is linoleic acid – this is a major constituent of such vegetable oils as corn oil, sunflower and safflower oils. However, linoleic acid has little biological activity, and in order to be of use to the body it must be metabolized (or converted) to gamma-linolenic acid (GLA). Studies suggest that a number of hyperactive and allergic children may be unable to metabolize essential fatty acids because they lack sufficient linoleic acid, or the necessary co-factors (zinc, B vitamins and vitamin C). (See Appendix 2.)

Some plant seeds contain GLA. It is found in the seeds of the evening primrose plant. Evening primrose oil, made from these seeds, is now widely available. For some conditions it is available on prescription through the NHS. (See also Appendix 2.)

The HACSG has found that supplements of zinc and other important co-factors such as vitamin B_6, nicotinamide and vitamin C, plus evening primrose oil are beneficial to hyperactive and allergic children, especially those suffering from abnormal thirst and children from 'atopic' families. (Atopic families are those in which eczema, asthma, hayfever and allergies are common.) It would seem likely that children who were not breast-fed may need this type of fat for a period of time to replenish cells that may have been deprived in the first nine months of life.

Warning: If the child is epileptic do not give evening primrose oil. Consult HACSG or Foresight for further advice.

MEALS

It is, of course, up to the individual family what foods are eaten at certain times of day, as this is partly a matter of convenience and individual preference. However, but a child going off to school without a good breakfast will find it more difficult to sit still and concentrate and learn.

Breakfast

The hyperactive child who has not been used to eating breakfast may at first not be very hungry in the morning. (This is mainly due to the lack of the B complex vitamins, zinc and vitamins C and E, and will soon improve if he is given supplements.) In the meantime it may only be possible to get him to drink. If he is not sensitive to cow's milk or goat's milk, try a milkshake. A banana milkshake with egg (from a guaranteed salmonella-free source) and honey makes a good sustaining breakfast. If he is not salicylate-sensitive, try fruit milkshakes made with stewed fruit, perhaps adding cashew or almond nut butter or avocado.

Later on you can try him on a wholegrain cereal, muesli or porridge, or a cooked breakfast (bacon and egg, or fish) and some raw fruit** or fruit juice**. (See pp. 33–36 for other suggestions.)

Try to avoid wheat cereal and wheat bread or toast at the same meal as it is important not to overload his system with wheat or dairy products to the exclusion of other foods. Raw fruit or vegetable at every meal is a good rule.

Lunch

School lunches vary enormously. Ask what the children have for lunch. If you are trying to avoid food additives, you may need to explain this. The more parents who say that their child should be kept on additive-free foods, the more the schools will get used to accommodating them. If the response is unsympathetic, ask if he can take a packed lunch.

Wholewheat sandwiches – cheese, marmite, hard-boiled egg – salad and nuts can be transported without difficulty, as can wholewheat cakes, biscuits and raw fruit. *Do not* make fish or meat sandwiches, as these can 'go off' in a warm building and cause serious illness.

The evening meal

This might be meat, fish or poultry with salad, or soup, followed by pudding.

Soup

Almost anything can go into soup, including a teaspoon of brewer's yeast, which will help increase the B vitamins. A bone broth base is rich in minerals.

Salads

As many raw ingredients as possible, e.g. sprouted seeds, raw mushrooms, raw cauliflower, shredded cabbage with nuts and grated carrot, mustard and cress, beetroot, celery, and permitted fruits.

Salad dressings

Oil, honey and lemon juice, yoghurt, soured cream, French dressing, mayonnaise.

Cakes and biscuits

These are far more nutritious when made with whole flour (see page 12). They can be made to rise by adding small quantities of bicarbonate of soda and cream of tartar, and by beating egg whites stiffly and folding them into the mixture (baking powder may contain additives – check the label).

Bread

You can make your own wholewheat bread, although in many areas you can buy good wholewheat bread.

Puddings

Crumbles, sponges, steamed puddings all taste better made with whole flour. Stewed fruit** and milk puddings – junket, custard, ice cream, milk jelly, rice, barley, sago, tapioca – can all be used to reduce the wheat content of the diet.

The evening meal should not contain too much wheat. Salad, soup (thickened with potato or yellow or green pea flour) and certain puddings can reduce the wheat content of the diet. So too can using a variety of flours (see p. 12).

The aim should be to provide a wide variety of cereals and starches.

Ideas for meals

The following pages set out specific menus for ten days, which are based on the whole food, additive-free principles we discussed earlier. They give a good picture of a balanced diet, avoiding repetitious use of wheat – even wholewheat! – every day. If he has a wheat cereal for breakfast, he has a different cereal for pudding – rice, for example, or sago – and has *Ryvita* for tea.

If he has egg, he only has it once in the day – preferably not more than 4–5 a week.

Jam is used sparingly – perhaps once in 4 days. Salads and raw fruit are used often if the child is not salicylate-sensitive.

Vegetables are rotated – leaf (cabbage, lettuce, Brussels sprouts etc.), root (turnip, carrot, parsnip, beetroot), flower (cauliflower, broccoli, calabrese), bulb (onions, and leeks), fruit (cucumbers**, marrow, pumpkin, courgette, tomatoes** and mushrooms.

Meats too, rotate – brown meat (beef, lamb, pork), white meat (poultry, rabbit), offal (heart, liver, kidneys, brain). Fish.

All types of cereal are brought into play – as well as wheat, rye (*Ryvita*), oats (pinhead and plain oatmeal), rice (brown, whole, ground and flaked and rice flour), polenta, barley (pearl barley), millet, buckwheat, sago, tapioca, peaflour. This makes it very easy to ring the changes.

Potato once a day is enough. If he has rice for lunch, he can have baked or mashed potato for supper.

Ideally, the more fruit and vegetables that can be home-grown the better. These can be completely fresh and free from contamination.

However, 'Pick-it-Yourself' and other organic market gardens and farms are now much more common.

The Foresight Association Branch Secretaries all keep a file of organic suppliers in their districts. In many cases farms can supply not only fruit and vegetables, but also wheat, meat and milk. One Foresight doctor has found that out of six 'wheat allergic' patients, four can eat organically grown wheat without reaction. It makes practical good sense to give the organic movement in this country all the support we can.

If you do not know of a local supplier, write, enclosing an S.A.E., to Foresight, marking the envelope 'Organic Produce Supplier'.

It can get to be *fun* planning a week's menu, balancing starch, protein and fruit and vegetable – getting in a raw fruit or vegetable every day, juggling with the cereals, the types of vegetables and the types of meat.

Try to avoid all white flour and refined sugar. Excess sugar, cakes, biscuits, sweets, chocolate, etc. can result in an increase in behavioural problems and can produce excessive thirst.

It is quite an intelligence test – I am sure you can pick holes in my menu – but you get the general idea!

Shop for small amounts of food, so there are not a lot of left-overs.

Of course, children have individual allergies and individual tastes and these must be accommodated – this is just a guide, not a set of rules!

Day 1
Breakfast
Oatmeal porridge
Poached egg on whole-
wheat toast
Fruit juice

Lunch
Rabbit with rice
Beans
Buckwheat pancake
with jam

Tea/Supper
Bone broth (pork bone)
with pearl barley
Macaroons
Mashed banana

Day 3
Breakfast
Museli with sultanas**
and apple**
Boiled egg with *Ryvita*
and butter

Lunch
Ox kidney and rice
Turnip
Sago pudding with
stewed apricots**

Day 2
Breakfast
Rice Krispies
Bacon (nitrate free) and sauté
potatoes
Fruit juice** or melon

Lunch
Scallops with cheese sauce
Bean sprouts
Mashed potato
Natural yoghurt with honey
and grapes**

Tea/Supper
Omelette
Tomato and cress salad
Wholewheat gingerbread
with nuts

Day 4
Breakfast
Millet porridge
Finnan haddock with rice

Lunch
Potatoes in Irish Stew with
pearl barley
Lamb chops
Broccoli
Baked banana
Milk jelly

Tea/Supper
Sausage (pork) and mash
Raw cabbage and grated
carrot salad
'Cow cake' with
sultanas** (see p. 40)

Day 5
Breakfast
Millet porridge
Dates wrapped in bacon
(nitrate free)
Ryvita, butter
and Marmite

Lunch
Pigeon
Roast parsnips
Leeks
Tapioca pudding

Tea/Supper
Herring roes
Grilled tomato**
Wholewheat shortbread
Baked potato

Day 7
Breakfast
Lamb's kidney and bacon
Fruit juice
Pineapple
Oatcakes with Marmite

Tea/Supper
Soup – bone broth with onion
and meat pieces
Wholewheat toast and jam
Prunes** or melon

Day 6
Breakfast
Prunes**
Egg and bacon (nitrate free)
Ryvita with molasses

Lunch
Lamb chop
Cabbage
Baked potato
Junket
Stewed apple** with honey

Tea/Supper
Fresh mackerel
Tomato and cress salad
Wholewheat bread and
butter, or cake

Day 8
Breakfast
Shredded Wheat
Sardines
Raw apple**

Lunch
Chicken with rice
Carrot
Custard
Jam tart (wholewheat)

Tea/Supper
Potato with cheese
Lettuce and cucumber**
Tapioca walnut pudding

Day 9
Breakfast
Millet porridge
Scrambled egg and bacon
Fruit juice
Orange**

Lunch
Potatoes boiled in
jackets
Liver, tomatoes** and
onions
Wholewheat sponge
pudding

Tea/Supper
Chicken bone broth with
peas, or lentils, pea flour
Ryvita with peanut
butter
Junket or mashed banana

Lunch
Haddock Pie
Cauliflower
Rice pudding with prunes**

Tea/Supper
Baked potato
Beetroot and yoghurt salad
Mashed banana
'Cow cake'

Day 10
Breakfast
Rice Krispies
Herring
Raw pear

Lunch
Baked potatoes
Minced beef
Marrow**
Tapioca
Bon Maman Cherry
Compote

Tea/Supper
Baked beans** with
mushrooms on wholewheat
toast
Polenta pudding

The HACSG provides a 'shopping basket' list with every *HACSG Handbook*. This list is updated every three months, as necessary.

Things to avoid

Coloured toothpaste, soap, bath bubbles, etc.

Antacids, quinine sulphate (in some cough mixtures)

Aspirin-based products.** *Paracetamol* may be given for headaches but should be kept to a minimum.
Tartrazine (E102) and other artificial colourings and/or sweeteners may be present in children's medicines. It is very important to check with your GP or pharmacist that your child's medicines are free from these additives.

Septrin and Calpol. We have had reports that Calpol and the antibiotic Septrin produce a strong reaction in some children.

RECIPES

Wholewheat bread

3lb (1.3kg) 100 per cent wholewheat stoneground flour
3 teaspoonsful salt (preferably sea salt)
1 oz (25g) fresh yeast (or ½ oz [12g] dried yeast soaked
    in 2 tablespoonsful of warm water till softened)
1 teaspoonful dark brown sugar
1 tablespoonful vegetable oil (optional) ·
Approx. 1½ pints (900ml) of warm water (just hand
    hot)

Makes 5 1-lb loaves

1. Put flour and salt into a large mixing bowl, and stand it somewhere to get warm, if necessary over a bowl of hot water.
2. Mix yeast and sugar and 2 tablespoonsful warm water and leave in a warm place (an airing cupboard will do) for about 10 minutes till covered with small bubbles.
3. Make a hollow in the flour and pour in frothy yeast and oil, if used.
4. Add 1½ pints (900ml) warm water and mix well together to make a smooth dough. If the dough is too dry to bind together, add just a little more water and mix in well. The dough should be slightly softer than pastry but not as moist as for fruit cake.
5. Put the dough on a well-floured board and knead well, turning the dough round and picking up the edge and pressing this into the centre. Keep on turning the dough and pressing new sides into the centre for about 5 minutes.
6. Put the dough back into the bowl, cover with a damp cloth and leave in warm place until almost doubled in size (about 30–45 minutes).
7. Preheat oven to 450°F/230°C (Gas Mark 8).
8. Turn risen dough out onto floured board and knead again lightly.
9. Divide into five equal pieces and knead each into shape to fit 1-lb tins, which should be greased and warmed. If preferred, make four loaves and a batch of rolls.
10. Cover with a cloth and leave in a warm (not hot) place until the dough is about ½ inch above the top of the tin (usually about 30 minutes).
11. Bake at 450°F/230°C (Gas Mark 8) for approximately 30–35 minutes. The loaves should be lightly browned on top, and sound hollow when tapped on the bottom. Rolls will take a shorter time.
12. Put on rack to cool.

Basic cake mixture

This basic mixture will make any type of cake, with nuts, permitted fruits, etc. It will also make a good steamed pudding. If tolerated, chocolate, cinnamon, spices etc. may be added for flavour.

4oz (100g) wholewheat flour (a combination of other flours such as whole rice and cornflour)
4oz (100g) butter (or corn oil)
4oz (100g) raw sugar (Barbados or Muscavado)
2 eggs
1 level teaspoonful of baking powder (aluminium- and colour-free)

Cream the butter and sugar and beat well. Add the eggs with a little flour, then gradually fold in the rest of the flour.

For a light sponge, add a heaped teaspoonful of cornflour. Put this on the weighing scales first and then make the flour up to 4oz (100g). Bake at 400°F/200°C (Gas Mark 6) for 15 minutes. Cook for a few minutes longer than for a 'white' recipe.

Basic biscuit mixture

1oz (25g) cornflour
7oz (190g) wholewheat flour
4oz (100g) butter
4oz (100g) raw sugar
1 egg
(Can be flavoured with grated lemon rind or cinnamon if neither affects the child adversely.)

Cream the butter and sugar and beat well. Add egg with a little flour, then gradually fold in rest. Roll out the mixture on a board. Cut into shapes, put on a greased oven sheet and bake in a moderate oven 350°F/180°C (Gas Mark 4) for 10 minutes. Remove and allow to cool, and then replace in the oven for a further 10 minutes, to give a crisper biscuit.

Shortbread

8oz (200g) wholewheat flour
2oz (50g) raw sugar
4oz (100g) butter
(If he is not salicylate-sensitive, use 6oz (150g) flour – wholewheat or a mixture of 2oz (50g) cornflour and 4oz (100g) whole rice flour – and 2oz (50g) ground almonds.)

Work sugar into the flour. Then work butter in with the fingers. Press down into buttered sponge tin. Prick centre with a fork, and mark round the edge with a fork. Cook at 350°F/180°C (Gas Mark 4) for about 40 minutes. Do not remove from the tin until cold.

Cow cake

6oz (150g) rolled oats
4oz (100g) butter
4oz (100g) raw cane sugar

Mix all ingredients together, press into a baking tin and cook at 350°F/180°C (Gas Mark 4) for about 25 minutes. Cut into fingers while still hot.

Gingerbread

¼ level teaspoonful bicarbonate of soda
Pinch of salt
1oz (25g) shredded almonds (substitute equivalent of
    flour if child is salicylate-sensitive)
2oz (50g) raw sugar
½–1 teaspoonful ginger   } Find out if child is
½–1 teaspoonful cinnamon   } sensitive to these
1 handful of sultanas if tolerated
1 handful of cashew nuts (optional)
4oz (100g) wholewheat flour
1oz (25g) pinhead oatmeal
2oz (50g) molasses
3oz (75g) butter
1 egg
1 dessertspoonful of water, if required, to mix
1 teaspoonful sunflower seed oil

Mix together all the dry ingredients. Melt together the butter, treacle and mix in with dry ingredients. Add beaten egg. Cook at 350°F/180°C (Gas Mark 4) for about 15 minutes, then turn down and leave in for a further 20 minutes. This gingerbread improves with keeping.

Scones

4oz (100g) wholewheat flour
1 tablespoonful of wheat germ
1oz (25g) butter
½oz (12½g) raw cane sugar
½ level teaspoonful bicarbonate of soda
1 egg
1 teaspoonful of milk (approximately)
Sultanas or currants if tolerated

Put dry ingredients into a bowl and rub in the fat. Add the egg and the milk and mix to a dough. Roll the dough into balls and pat to approximately ½ inch flat. Pop in a hot oven – 450°F/230°C (Gas Mark 8) – for about 8–10 minutes.

Gluten-free sponge cake

4oz (100g) butter
4oz (100g) raw sugar
2 eggs
½oz (12½g) cornflour
2oz (50g) rice flour
2oz (50g) potato or sago flour
Pinch of salt
1 rounded teaspoonful of home-made baking powder

Cream the butter and sugar and beat well. Add the eggs. Mix the dry ingredients in bowl and then fold in gradually. Bake in greased sandwich tins in a preheated oven – 400°F/200°C (Gas Mark 6) for 15 minutes.

Gluten-free scones

4 heaped tablespoonsful *Jubilee* bread mix
1½ heaped tablespoonsful gluten-free muesli base
1 rounded tablespoonful raw sugar
½ teaspoonful bicarbonate of soda
2oz (50g) butter or margarine
1–2 tablespoonsful milk

Put dry ingredients in a bowl and mix well. Rub in butter, and mix in milk to make a damp dough. Form into little rounds, place on a greased baking tray and bake in a hot oven – 400°F/200°C (Gas Mark 6) – for 8–9 minutes.

Gluten-free little cakes

4oz (100g) butter
4oz (100g) raw sugar
1½oz (37½g) yellow pea flour
1½oz (37½g) brown rice flour
1½oz (37½g) polenta
2 eggs
1 level teaspoonful cream of tartar
½ level teaspoonful bicarbonate of soda
Nuts or permitted fruits and flavourings

Follow method for sponge cake and divide the mixture into patty pans. Bake in a preheated oven 400°F/200°C (Gas Mark 6) for 15 minutes.

Notes

1. Organically-grown vegetables are available from some health food stores. The Organic Food Service, The Soil Association and The Foresight Association can all provide addresses of places which sell organically-grown food (see Useful Addresses).
2. See note 1 above for details of sources of meat from organic farms.
3. See note 1.

CHAPTER 3

ALLERGIES

In recent years, allergy is believed to have surpassed infection
as a major cause of illness. Although sensitivity to
substances such as pollen and animal fur has long been
recognized, the wider implications of chemical pollution and
food additives are now beginning to be understood. Contact
dermatitis from washing powders and other skin irritations
such as rashes, eczema, psoriasis and sweating are old news.
Chemical irritation of the mucous membranes leads to
mouth ulcers, sneezing, asthma, hay fever – which takes the
form of running eyes and nose, or stomach discomfort, colitis,
and/or bloating. Diarrhoea occurs in coeliac disease. What is
new is that allergic reactions can cause a whole group of mental and emotional problems, a common one for example being
simply a feeling of continual fatigue. The child in chronic discomfort is more likely to be restless, whiney and hyperactive.

Medical people argue as to whether these adverse reactions to foods and inhaled substances should be called allergic
reactions, intolerances or food sensitivities. Whatever name
is given to the problem, the solution is the same – once it has
been identified reliably, avoid the substance.

Allergies and hyperactivity

Almost any allergen can cause hyperactivity in a susceptible child.[1] Hyperactive children have highly sensitive nervous systems, which would explain why in a family which eats the same food only one child becomes a victim. Children who are allergically sensitive to food are often also sensitive to inhaled allergens. They might perhaps only be *seasonally* hyperactive at the time that grass and trees are pollenating. Other common allergens are cigarette smoke, car and diesel exhaust fumes, animal dandruff, effluent from North Sea gas and hydrocarbons from plastics. Where possible the suspected source should be removed for a short period to confirm or deny the connection. Allergic reactions are more common in the poor feeder who may have nutritional deficiencies which lead to inadequacies of the immune system and in the child who was given artificial feeding at an early age.

HOW DO ALLERGIES START?

Nutrient deficiencies in the mother

An American study[2] on cats has produced evidence to suggest that trace mineral deficiencies in the mother produced kittens with allergies.

In a study at Charing Cross Hospital[3] in London, Dr Ellen Grant found that, in adults, smoking and the contraceptive pill increased the chances of food allergy. Smoking is known to increase levels of cadmium and lead and decrease levels of zinc, and vitamin B complex, C and E. The pill is known to decrease levels of zinc, manganese, vitamins B_6, B_2, B_{12} and C. By increasing excretion of vitamin B_6 in the urine, zinc deficiency would reduce levels of nicotinamide (made in the intestine with the help of B_6 and B_2). Plasma vitamin A could also be compromised, as zinc is necessary for the conversion for the conversion of beta-carotene to plasma vitamin A.

It is, therefore, possible that children born to women who smoke or who have recently discontinued the pill will be lacking in these nutrients and therefore more allergy prone, as these essential nutrients are needed for the production of enzymes necessary to metabolize food correctly, and for optimal adrenal function.

The HACSG Database on 700 plus hyperactive children shows that 72 per cent of these children were hyperactive *in utero*. Research also shows that babies can be sensitized to cow's milk intolerance *in utero*. Mothers with undiagnosed milk allergy may drink a lot of milk during pregnancy.

Many of these babies have wriggled so much that they are born with their umbilical cord wound round their bodies and necks several times. An American researcher says this is not likely to cause mental delay, but is sufficient to cause some learning difficulties.

A Health Visitor reporting in the *Nursing Mirror* says that hyperactivity may start *in utero* as early as 18 weeks' gestation. At 20 weeks the foetus responds readily to sounds and activity by tossing and turning endlessly, often to such an extent that mothers have asked if the unborn baby is in distress!

A high proportion of these hyperactive children suffer from severe colic. Research from the US suggests that a cow milk protein, Bovine IgG, present in infant formula and also passed to breastfed babies when mothers eat dairy foods, causes infant colic. Analysis consistently showed higher Bovine IgG in the breast milk of mothers of 'colicky' babies. Sixty per cent of these babies improved when mother avoided cow's milk.

The HACSG Database also shows that a large percentage of these children are born into 'atopic' families (those in which allergies are more common). Many mothers of these children suffer from migraine, and families show hay fever, rhinitis, asthma and eczema. Arthritis, diabetes and thyroid problems have also been recorded.

Early feeding habits

Adverse reactions may be brought on by too early an introduction of cow's milk, sugar, supplements such as orange juice or fish-liver oils, vitamin drops containing artificial colouring and flavouring, and even solid feeding. A baby's immature digestive tract is prepared only for breast milk in the first five to six months of life.

In a research study (*Lancet*, June 1992) at St Mary's Hospital on the Isle of Wight, the conclusion was that 'the reduction in exposure of high risk infants to allergens in food and in housedust *substantially lowers the frequency of allergic reactions* in infancy ... parents' smoking contributes greatly to the development of allergic disorders during infancy and should be avoided.'

Food additives

Another problem is, as we have seen, the introduction of 'foreign bodies' into our diet. 'Food additives' are, in reality, anything but food – 'non-food' additives would be a better description! According to Dr Ben Feingold, the body may detoxify these additives by coating them in a substance the body tolerates, such as zinc, and then passing them out via the liver or kidneys. Thus, over a period of time, they squander body reserves of zinc or other protective nutrients.

Nutritional deficiencies in the child

The HACSG has found that, due to undiagnosed food intolerance (often cow's milk/dairy foods), the child may suffer quite severe colic, which may go on for several weeks or longer. The lining of the intestine (gut) can break down and become more permeable (this is known as leaky gut syndrome), letting substances into the blood which should have been broken down before passing through the intestinal wall.

Unfortunately, if this occurs, nutrients from food (or supplements) will not be fully absorbed. It is therefore crucial that colic is dealt with quickly, before too much damage is done.

If breast milk cannot be made available, diluted goat's milk or soya formula may be preferable to cow's milk formulae. However, clearly a national policy of making it easier for mothers to be with their babies for the first nine months needs to be more clearly defined and supported.

Pollution

Another problem is believed to be that lead, chlorine, North Sea gas, flouride and other pollutants inhibit the production of enzymes, as does a paucity of the nutrients the body needs. Indoor gas boilers can cause considerable pollution.

These theories do not, in fact, conflict. The baby in the womb whose trace mineral nourishment has been minimal, is the baby from the poorly-nourished mother in whom lactation may easily fail. Once the mother finds herself short of breast milk, she must resort to unnatural and unsuitable substances to try to satisfy the infant's demands. Cow's milk, sugar, orange juice, fish-liver oil and an assortment of cereals may shortly assault the infant's delicate digestive tract, causing metabolic chaos and possibly malabsorption.

The injured intestinal tract may allow undigested particles of food to pass through into the circulating blood: vital trace minerals may not be absorbed, vital intestinal flora may be superseded by unpropitious flora which may encourage the growth of unwanted bacteria, which in turn may sap the baby's strength. Vitamin and mineral deficiencies may then abound.

Added to these problems is the fact that with every breath the child takes he may inhale lead, traffic exhaust fumes, cigarette smoke, hydrocarbons, outgassing from plastics, and effluent from factories and/or North Sea gas. With every mouthful he eats or drinks, he may take in lead, copper and/or aluminium contamination, a plethora of chemical additives, and a number of foods to which his body has become sensitized as a result of too-early weaning. It is hardly surprising he has a problem!

POSITIVE ACTION

1. Introduce a good, wholefood diet of foods he can tolerate (we discussed this in Chapter 2).
2. Remove toxic metals and supplement necessary trace elements (see Chapter 4).
3. Identify and eliminate substances he cannot tolerate.

Identifying food allergies

If, after having introduced a good wholefood diet, the child is not very much improved in eight weeks, it is worth going to some trouble to pinpoint possible allergies. Writing down everything your child has to eat or drink (including snacks) each day for seven days, and clearly noting any behavioural problems, aches/pains, crying, poor sleep patterns, etc., can be a very useful way of pinpointing foods or drinks which may be causing the problems.

Look back and see if you can remember when the hyperactivity/screaming/night-waking/diarrhoea/eczema/asthma or whatever started. If it was (as it so often is) when he was weaned off the breast onto cow's milk, and you suspect that your child may have an allergy or intolerance of cow's milk, *it is important that you seek professional advice*, either from your doctor, or community dietician (at the local hospital).

Eliminating cow's milk for a few weeks, and then re-introducing it again, may cause severe problems, if the child has an 'undiagnosed' intolerance to cow's milk.

If he was weaned early but seemed happy on the bottle, he may have adapted successfully to the cow's milk, and the next stumbling block may have been the introduction of cereals. If he was introduced to cereals before four-and-a-half to five months, he may well have had diarrhoea, or been restless, grizzly and unable to settle. If this continued, he may have a grain allergy. Citrus allergy, started by a bad reaction to orange juice, may also be easy to spot.

If the allergies seemed to develop later in life, when he was taking a wide variety of foods, then it may be more difficult to pinpoint the specific food or foods. Many children have three or four allergenic foods, a few have even more. Sometimes the reaction does not come for some hours, which makes it quite hard to identify, but with perseverance you can win through.

Keeping a food diary, this time for a few weeks, may be helpful. If the problem is something he only eats occasionally, such as chocolate, this method of detection will often be successful.

If your doctor is quite sympathetic it is possible to get tests done, and sometimes these are very helpful (and will probably confirm what you already suspected), but only a limited number of foods will be tested, and none of the ways of testing is 100 per cent reliable.

The other option is to try the child on a rotation diet (given on p. 53) for two or three weeks. It is a great bore, but it really does show up allergies as nothing else can. The child takes each food once a week only, and the reaction will be sharper as the child will have gone without this food for a week. (The other alternative is the 'Caveman 'Diet' on p. 99).

While nobody wants to restrict a young child's diet unnecessarily, the benefits of freeing the child from the detrimental effects of the food he is sensitive to, make it worth removing the offending food from his diet completely for at least several years, in some cases maybe for life.

If a major food is to be excluded from the diet, it is important to check to see which vitamins and minerals would have been present in this food, and to compensate accordingly. For example, milk is high in minerals and vitamins A and D; so if he is not to have milk, he will need plenty of bone broth, possibly bonemeal or dolomite tablets, and plenty of green vegetables. If he can take fish-liver oil, this will compensate for the vitamins. If he has to go without grain he will need all the minerals, the B complex vitamins and vitamin E. If your child cannot eat wheat or tolerate cow products, you may feel your problems have only just begun. On p. 100 we give suggestions for milk-free and gluten-free diets, and if your doctor is sympathetic he or she may put you in touch with a dietitian who will be able to give you further help.

Coeliac disease

In cases of coeliac disease (malabsorption due to sensitivity to the gluten grains – wheat, oats, barley and rye) there has usually been a history of loose stools, or big bulky stools, probably passed several times a day since early childhood. Sometimes these stools are very pale; sometimes they are full of undigested food; sometimes the child has long bouts of diarrhoea which are quite difficult to stop – especially when teething.

The child is thin, hyperactive, easily tired, very prone to tears and tantrums, talkative and overexcitable. Pant-and bed-wetting is common and sleeping is usually poor. He may complain of abdominal pain or rectal cramp.

A good idea is to give the child a diet which contains no flour products and cereals for about four weeks to see if the symptoms abate. If so, it is worth asking your GP to arrange the child to be screened for coeliac disease.

A ROTATED DIET FOR THE DETECTION OF ALLERGY

The rotated diet on p. 53 is designed to give each specific food only one day in seven. The diet eliminates the most common allergens – cow's milk, grains and eggs – also all stimulants such as coffee, tea, chocolate and sugar.

Where possible all four foods listed should be taken at each meal and no drink should be taken except the juice of the day and water. All foods must be boiled in plain water, steamed, grilled or cooked in the oven in a covered dish. No fats, oils or gravies are to be used. During the trial period no food other than those listed may be taken at all.

During the first week of the diet adverse reactions may take place due to the withdrawal of cow's milk, etc. if these are allergenic substances. For a few days the reactions may be quite strong – akin to the alcoholic withdrawal in the first few days of abstinence.

The food can be taken in various ways. Tuesday's breakfast could be grilled pork slice; lunch a pork chop; supper slices from a pork joint. On Wednesdays, breakfast could be

A rotated diet

Monday	Tuesday	Wednesday	Thursday	Friday	Saturday	Sunday
Chicken	Pork	Lamb	Turkey	Fish	Rabbit	Duck
Banana	Sago	Brown rice	Maize (sweetcorn)	Millet	Lentils	Potato
Pineapple	Dates	Orange	Cornflower	Millet flakes	Green beans	Tomato
Beetroot	Apple	Grapefruit	Leeks	Cabbage	Peas	Aubergine
Spinach	Pear	Satsuma	Onions	Savoy cabbage	Black-eyed beans	Cucumber
Swiss chard	Lettuce	Mandarin	Asparagus	Brussels	Broad beans	Marrow
Pineapple juice	Endive	Lime	Chives	Sprouts	Mung bean shoots	Melon
	Chicory	Carrot	Grapes	Broccoli	Plums	Tomato juice
	Artichoke	Celery	Sultanas	Cauliflower	Peaches	
	Sunflower seeds	Parsnip	Grape juice	Kohlrabi	Apricot	
	Apple juice	Parsley		Swedes	Cherry	
		Orange or grapefruit juice		Avocado	Prunes	
				Figs	Prune juice	
				Water		

lamb's kidneys: lunch could be a lamb chop and the evening meal could be lamb's liver. Please remember that if your child is salicylate-sensitive the menus will have to be altered accordingly.

Unfinished food of the day should be put in the freezer for the following week. If only fruit and vegetables which will be consumed on the day are bought, this removes temptation for the following day. The child may be more hungry than usual, however, and it is important to have enough food available.

The diet will have ensured six days without the offending food so the reaction to the allergen will probably be fairly immediate and take the form of a runny or stuffed-up nose, headache, stomach pain, feeling of bloatedness, extreme lethargy or hyperactivity, irritability, etc. The day this occurs can be marked on the diet sheet. It is then possible to test the foods eaten on this day one at a time.

Having thus worked out a basic diet of 'safe' foods, it will then be possible to test common allergens, such as eggs, the gluten grains – wheat, oats, barley, rye – and other fruits. After three weeks' abstinence the reaction may be strong, so at first only a small quantity of the substance should be given. If the reaction is very severe, a teaspoonful of bicarbonate of soda in water will help to alleviate the symptoms.

After an adverse reaction a return to known safe foods for a few days will be necessary before testing for another possible allergen. After a few weeks it should be possible to identify all food allergies in this way.

N.B. Retesting cow's milk should only be done under medical supervision.

IDENTIFYING INHALED ALLERGENS

Again detective work is needed. The types of questions you may need to ask are:

Is he worse in the winter? If so, could it be your gas fire?

Does he react more in heavy traffic than in the park or indoors?

Does he 'go silly' after playing with the cat or dog?

Is he worse in certain rooms where there are plastic-covered chairs/a coal fire?

The HACSG has found the following inhaled allergens commonly affect children: household cleaners and polishes, aerosols, hair sprays and perfumes, felt-tip pens, fly killers, solid air fresheners and insecticides and coloured bubble bath. Once you know the type of thing to look for the picture may be clarified surprisingly quickly. 'He's always been really bad in the car – especially in the town I've noticed'; 'When he's been with the horses, he seems to go beserk and then fall asleep'; 'He was so much better all summer, then it all started again in September – it must have been when we started using the gas fire again', are the type of observations which help to pinpoint the problem.

IDENTIFYING VERY DIFFICULT CASES

The conventional 'skin tests' and 'sublingual (under the tongue) drop' tests have their uses with very difficult cases. There are some excellent doctors working with allergy on both sides of the Atlantic, and if spending a few weeks in careful observation and manipulating the diet fails to come up with a clear-cut answer, it is worth seeking a doctor who can help with the detection work. (HACSG and Foresight can supply addresses, see Useful Addresses.)

'GROWING OUT' OF ALLERGIES

As the child's system is rested from dealing with foods to which he reacts badly, the intestinal tract may heal and the beneficial intestinal flora increase in number, so that the child's general health is improved. Supplements of vitamin A, B complex and zinc help both this healing process and the development of the enzyme systems because, as the body level of beneficial trace minerals increases, 'enemies' such as lead will be excreted which will improve the chances of enzyme activity. This is why the 'allergies' may be 'grown out of' as the child's health improves.

With the coeliac child, evidence to date seems to suggest that the problem is life-long, but with other less virulent allergies, it may be possible to reintroduce the foods after a year or so – perhaps in small quantities and at stated intervals only. This will be a matter for you and your child to discuss and observe together. The older children get, the easier it is for them to co-operate. At eight or nine they can be surprisingly wise about their own reactions. If there is a bad reaction, however, this should be noted and the food discontinued again. When the episode is over it helps to discuss the way the food/fumes etc. affected him and to draw his attention to the connection. In this way your child will become involved in his health problem and can start to play a positive part in treating it.

Notes

1. 'One in five children has a food allergy or intolerance and prevalence is growing, nutrition experts have warned. Speaking at the Food, Children and Health conference at the Royal Society of Medicine in January, consultant dietitian Mabel Blades said that estimated incidence of food allergy intolerance among young children is between 2 and 20 per cent. But many children can remain undiagnosed, and so do not get the specialist help they need. "A large number of conditions are related to food allergy and food intolerance. Health professionals need to increase their awareness and refer to families for advice," she said.' Heather Welford (1997) *Health Visitor*, 70, 3, p.91.

2. Dr Frank Pottenger of the Price Pottenger Association, PO Box 2614, La Mesa, California 92041.

3. See Dr Ellen Grant (1979) Food allergies and migraine *The Lancet* 1, 1, p.966; (1981) article in *The International Journal of Environmental Studies* 17, 1, p.57–66.

CHAPTER 4

HEAVY METAL TOXICITIES, TRACE MINERAL DEFICIENCIES AND HAIR ANALYSIS

We live in a constantly changing and increasingly hazardous environment. Many pollutants which the adult body may have learned to cope with, detoxify and discard, are a danger to the health and development of small children, so the modern parent has had to become increasingly vigilant to protect the child's well-being. It is now part of our job as parents to become informed about harmful substances children are likely to come in contact with, and to take positive action.

HEAVY METAL TOXICITIES

A number of important developments in lead research have contributed to the body of evidence linking lead levels in children tested in several industrialized countries to behavioural problems and IQ deficits ... It is generally accepted that children are particularly at risk from lead exposure because of the specific metabolic conditions of childhood, and the vulnerability of the developing nervous system.[1]

In her work with 'mentally disturbed' children,[2] the Californian paediatrician Dr Elizabeth Lodge-Rees has found them to be disadvantaged both emotionally and mentally not only by a high body-burden of lead but also by cadmium, mercury, aluminium and excess copper. She writes: 'These children may have many minor health problems, allergic syndromes, hyperactivity, dyslexia, learning difficulties or in many cases just poor school records and a persistent inability to "fit in" with the day-to-day demands of normal life.'

Lead

The lead content of the air we breathe rose sharply up until 1987 due partly to the higher lead content of petrol and partly to the increase in car ownership in Britain.

Studies from this country, the US, Australia and Switzerland correlated the high body-lead with hyperactivity, learning difficulties, congenital anomaly of the central nervous system, stillbirth and cancer.

Professor Lawther in the late 1970s headed a group of government scientists who brought out a report entitled *Lead and Health*[3] which queried the validity of all these studies. In November 1980, Professor D. Bryce-Smith of Reading University and Dr R. Stephens of Birmingham University published a reply entitled *Lead or Health*.[4] We suggest parents who would like to study the question for themselves read both these reports.

In the 1980s it was calculated that 76,000 tonnes of lead were emitted from car exhausts every year. This lead circulated in the air we breathed and the dust in our houses, and landed on food crops, soil, water and grazing land. Beyond question, the worst areas of lead pollution were the urban areas where the traffic was thickest,[5] and there were more hyperactive children in towns and cities than in rural areas.

In the US, a Dr Billick did a study showing that the blood levels of lead in city children rose and fell with the seasonal variation in the amount of leaded petrol sold at petrol stations.

In 1987 lead-free petrol was made available, at a slightly reduced price. No serious publicity was given by Government or medical pundits about how necessary it was, nor were pointers given on how to adapt car engines for its use. However, about one-third of the population started to use it, and the work of Dr Stephen Davies of Biolab shows that the lead levels in the general population started to reduce. It seemed hopeful that lead pollution was a problem that was on the way out. Sadly, although the levels in children have lessened, the pollution has only been reduced, not eliminated entirely.

It would be within the Government's power either to adjust taxation to make a significant difference in the price of leaded petrol compared to unleaded to eliminate leaded petrol by making it illegal or at the very least to insist leaded petrol was sold only to people whose cars could not be adapted.

Europe is asking for lead-free air by 1999. The UK is asking for an exemption to this. We are the only country to be doing so.

Traffic fumes are not the only source of lead in the environment, however. A number of households in this country have lead levels in the drinking water above that permitted by the World Health Organization. Lead in the drinking water had been correlated by Dr Michael Moore of Glasgow with mental retardation in babies. The higher the lead in the maternal drinking water, the greater the degree of mental retardation in the baby.

Flaking leaded-paint is frequently quoted as a source of lead in small children. This seems unlikely as not many mothers allow their children to eat paint continuously! But in rare cases, if decoration is in a very bad state of repair, dust from this type of paint might be a source of lead.

Without doubt the most widespread source of lead in children remains the lead in petrol – either inhaled directly from traffic fumes or from contaminated food.

Children with dark skins may absorb toxic metals more readily, possibly due to difficulties with calcium metabolism.

Copper

In soft-water areas the copper used in plumbing may leach into the drinking water. In some areas the water contains both lead and copper, the lead having come from the pipes under the road leading to the house and/or lead-glazed mains. Where the lead pipe leading to the house joins the copper pipe there is a type of electrical charge that causes the copper to leach lead. Particularly at risk are soft water areas where the water is acid as a result of the acid, peaty-type soil. This acidity tends to leach metal from the plumbing into the water. Unless the tap is run well beforehand, the baby having an early morning bottle is especially vulnerable because the kettle will be filled with water that has stood in the pipe overnight, and therefore contains a greater amount of both lead and copper than any other water drunk subsequently during the day.

Copper sulphate is used in swimming pools to kill algae, so if a child has a high copper hair analysis (see page 64) after swimming regularly in such a pool, a hair analysis reading could be false. Another sample should be checked six weeks after he has stopped swimming.

Copper is an essential mineral and any deficiency is detrimental.

Aluminium

The main source of aluminium is thought to be cooking pans and food cooked in foil. It is also found in substances such as *Coffee-Mate*, *Compliment*, *Gelusil* and indigestion tablets, and some salts and baking powders. As ever, read the labels on these products carefully and change to another brand if necessary. Very high aluminium levels have been found in people who use aluminium pressure-cookers and kettles. Children can get high levels from soya preparations and canned drinks. Some water is contaminated.

Cadmium

The main source of cadmium is parental cigarette smoke. Most hyperactive children have been found to improve when their parents stop smoking. Some cadmium can be obtained from alloys used in plumbing – yet again, soft water areas are more vulnerable.

Mercury

Mercury is said to be present in some fish, but as all seed wheat is dusted with mercury before sowing, it seems feasible that some may find its way into the drinking water where the rain has washed off the wheat fields into gullies and thence to the rivers. There is little that can be done about this. There is no reason to stop eating fish because it is not often contaminated. In any event, high mercury is not a frequent problem. Having said this, mercury dental amalgams should be avoided at all times, especially for children. There are alternatives available – ask your dentist.

Selenium

Rarely, over-high selenium can result from too-frequent use of selenium-containing shampoos, insufficient rinsing and use of such shampoos in the bath, etc. Detailed warnings are given on the bottles/wrappings of such shampoos. To avoid confused interpretation, the hair should not be tested until six weeks after discontinuing the use of a selenium-containing shampoo.

Selenium is an essential mineral, and deficiencies are far more common than over-high levels.

TRACE MINERAL IMBALANCE

Most minerals are better absorbed in the presence of vitamin C, the B complex vitamins and/or the essential fatty acids and vitamin E. Ideally it is best to give the mineral supplements as part of a vitamin and mineral supplementation programme.

The following vitamins should be supplied with the minerals:

calcium	vitamin D
magnesium	nicotinamide; B_6 and D
iron	vitamin C
copper	vitamin A
manganese	choline, B_6, pantothenate, biotin, folate, evening primrose oil, vitamin E
zinc	vitamin B_6, evening primrose oil, vitamin E
chromium	vitamin B_1 and nicotinamide
selenium	vitamin E

Vitamin B_{12} can be used alone to counteract cobalt deficiency.

Low sodium and potassium levels

It is often helpful to give vitamins A, C and E and B complex, particularly pantothenic acid and nicotinamide. These vitamins assist the adrenal glands to function and this in turn helps to combat the tendency to allergic syndromes. Stressed adrenal function can lead to sodium/potassium imbalance.

Junomac supplement

Junamac (see p. 27) provides calcium, magnesium, manganese, zinc and chromium with vitamins A, B, C, D and E, among other nutrients. It does not contain artificial colourings, preservatives, gluten, sugar or cane products. *Junamac* has been designed so that the correct supplement is one tablet per stone in bodyweight. It is suitable for children up to six stone in weight.

Essential fatty acids can be taken as capsules or drops, as can vitamin K. Zinc drops are available containing 5mg zinc, 1mg manganese and 10mg B_6 per drop.

Biocare do a range of drops including a multi-vitamin formula and mineral combinations.

Iron deficiency

If iron levels are just slightly low, raisins** soaked in lemon juice all day and eaten in the evening are a good source of iron. It is best to give iron in the evenings. Other minerals should be given at breakfast for maximum absorption.

Brewer's yeast

Cheaper, but less detailed supplementation, can be given with brewer's yeast (for those who are *not* yeast sensitive) and halibut-liver oil, either the liquid or in capsules. This, however, does not supply evening primrose oil or vitamin E, which have been found to be so helpful.

For more about evening primrose oil, please see Appendix 2.

Hair analysis

One method of screening to get an indication of whether a child has a high level of toxic metals and/or deficiencies of essential minerals is by hair analysis.

To obtain a hair sample, one tablespoonful of hair should be taken from the back of the head. It can be taken in small snippets from different places, so in most cases it will not be obvious that it has been cut at all. The sample should be taken from as close to the scalp as possible and each tuft should be not longer than 1 inch. Send an S.A.E. to either the HACSG or the Foresight Association requesting the application forms for a hair analysis. While treating for metal toxicities and/or deficiencies of trace minerals, the hair should be tested every four months.

There are a few typical patterns for hyperactivity that turn up time and again on the hair analyses (see Figures 1–4, beginning on page 66).

Poor Diet
The first and easiest to recognize is the pattern of a child who has been on an inadequate diet and probably had a very poor appetite, except for sweets and sugary 'junk' food. This pattern will often show low levels of trace minerals –

magnesium, iron, copper, zinc, manganese, chromium, selenium and cobalt – right across the board. If there are no over-high levels of toxic metals present, these children will respond to a diet rich in essential nutrients – whole grains, raw fruit and vegetables, a course of *Junamac* and other minerals as suggested.

	Results (mg/kg)	Recommended Values (mg/kg)
Calcium:	209	400
Magnesium:	31	35
Potassium:	61	75
Iron:	29	30
Chromium:	0.47	0.8
Cobalt:	0.20	0.25
Copper:	14	20
Manganese:	0.56	1.5
Nickel:	0.72	0.8
Selenium:	1.02	2.25
Zinc:	93	185
		Threshold values
		(levels above this are considered toxic) (mg/kg)
Aluminium:	1.64	2.5
Cadmium:	0.08	0.25
Mercury:	0.02	0.4
Lead:	1.14	1.0

Figure 1: Hair analysis of 11-year-old Child A suffering from apathy, fatigue, bruising, dyslexia, learning difficulties, memory loss, poor appetite, sensitivity to light and noise, underweight. Note deficiencies in most major minerals. [6]

	Results (mg/kg)	Recommended Values (mg/kg)
Calcium:	369	400
Magnesium:	38	35
Potassium:	74	75
Iron:	36	30
Chromium:	1.09	0.8
Cobalt:	0.29	0.25
Copper:	18	20
Manganese:	1.18	1.5
Nickel:	0.76	0.8
Selenium:	2.75	2.25
Zinc:	217	185
		Threshold values (mg/kg)
Aluminium:	2.91	2.5
Cadmium:	0.07	0.25
Mercury:	0.07	0.4
Lead:	3.01	1.0

Figure 2: Child A after 5½ months on supplementation. Note increase in all mineral levels, to approaching or well within recommended values. Note also body is cleansing itself of (throwing out) toxic metals, not visible in the previous chart.

	Results (mg/kg)	Recommended Values (mg/kg)
Calcium:	214	400
Magnesium:	30	35
Potassium:	82	75
Iron:	34	30
Chromium:	0.46	0.8
Cobalt:	0.21	0.25
Copper:	14	20
Manganese:	0.33	1.5
Nickel:	0.52	0.8
Selenium:	0.92	2.25
Zinc:	114	185
		Threshold values (mg/kg)
Aluminium:	5.99	2.5
Cadmium:	0.02	0.25
Mercury:	0.02	0.4
Lead:	4.72	1.0

Figure 3: Hair analysis of Child B, suffering from dental decay, diarrhoea, eczema, hyperactivity, learning difficulties, migraine, underweight. Note shortages of many essential minerals, and high levels of lead and aluminium.

	Results (mg/kg)	Recommended Values (mg/kg)
Calcium:	315	400
Magnesium:	36	35
Potassium:	71	75
Iron:	35	30
Chromium:	0.99	0.8
Cobalt:	0.19	0.25
Copper:	20	20
Manganese:	1.14	1.5
Nickel:	0.72	0.8
Selenium:	2.19	2.25
Zinc:	156	185
		Threshold values (mg/kg)
Aluminium:	1.02	2.5
Cadmium:	0.02	0.25
Mercury:	0.01	0.4
Lead:	0.96	1.0

Figure 4: Hair analysis of Child B after 6½ months on supplementation, including vitamin C and garlic. Note improvement in minerals and lowering of toxic metals, although calcium, manganese and zinc levels have a little way to go.

Malabsorption

Another common pattern is that of the child very low in minerals who does not respond even after four months of supplementation and dietary changes. This usually indicates malabsorption or infestation such as with threadworms. The latter can usually be detected just by asking the child if his bottom itches at night, and can be cured by powders prescribed by a GP. Pants, pyjamas, etc. should be washed in disinfectant and/or boiled to prevent re-infestation, and trousers should be washed or cleaned. Bedding and duvet covers will need to be cleaned as well.

Malabsorption may be due to coeliac disease or food allergy (see Chapter 3), or to a urinary tract infection, as this squanders nutrients as a result of diuresis (increased excretion of urine).

Toxic metals

Low mineral patterns may be seen in combination with a high toxic metal pattern, as a low level of zinc and/or manganese tends to make the child more prone to accumulating toxic metals, and high levels of lead etc. can drive manganese out of the body. The toxic metals can be cleansed from the body with vitamin C plus garlic.

If you require professional help, the HACSG and Foresight Association can supply addresses of doctors who are experienced in the field of heavy metal toxicity. Please enclose an S.A.E. with your request.

Water checks

If you have lead pipes or a lead tank, or if your water is very soft, it is probably worth asking your local water board to test the drinking water at tap-flow for lead, copper, cadmium and aluminium. If your water is above the WHO limit in any of the heavy metals, make an official complaint to your Water Board. It is important to use a water filter (either a *Kenwood* or *Boots* jug, or a 'whole house' filter). The carbon filter in the jug-type should be changed once a month. In heavily contaminated areas the water should be tested again after filtration.

If a child has not been taken to see his family doctor, the parents should do so before embarking on any self-help régime to ascertain the definite cause of any problems. Do bear in mind, however, that GPs are not trained in the effects of heavy metal toxicity, and may only have information on very gross mineral deficiency and contamination levels.

Notes

1. Jeannie Peterson, article in *Ambio* 8, 5.
2. Dr Elizabeth Lodge Rees, The Rees Medical Centre, 1511 North Carson Street, PO Box 2768, Carson City, Nevada 89701, USA.
3. *Lead and Health* (The Lawther Report) HMSO, 1980.
4. Professor D. Bryce-Smith *Lead or Health?* Conservation Society, 1980.
5. See I. H. Billick, A. S. Curran, D. R. Shier *Relation of pediatric blood levels to lead in gasoline* HUD Report (1979), The Environmental Research Group, Department of Housing and Urban Development, Washington DC 20410, USA.
6. Foresight – University of Surrey Research.

CHAPTER 5

DAY-TO-DAY MANAGEMENT OF THE HYPERACTIVE CHILD

Much has been written in recent years about the day-to-day management of the hyperactive child. However, most of the literature seems to be directed at the parents of the physiologically normal but 'difficult' child, rather than at the parents of the child whose biochemistry throws up a set of reactions which are entirely different from those of the normal child. So what follows are our suggestions, borne of the experience of living and coping with hyperactive children. While the hyperactivity persists (and treatment may take months rather than weeks) the most important thing is to keep conflict to a minimum and keep a constant check on the child's safety.

The anger and frustration a parent inevitably feels at times while coping with the completely atypical behaviour of the hyperactive child should be directed at those truly responsible. For example at the Government who, knowing the harm that airborne lead does to children, will still not eliminate the lead content of petrol; at the food manufacturers who still persist in using food colourants and flavouring banned in many other countries, and at the water authorities for providing contaminated water; and at the school caterers who (in some cases because of financial cutbacks) do not always encourage wholesome eating habits.

While the child is still hyperactive any reaction will be exaggerated. Where a normal child might not want to do something, the hyperactive child will refuse point blank and have a tantrum if pressed! Where a normal child may just pick up a bright toy, the hyperactive child may put it in his mouth, like a much younger child. Visitors, treats and outings that delight the normal child will result in overexcitement and uncontrollably wild behaviour with the hyperactive child.

The hyperactive child's parents must be constantly on the alert to avoid danger. If the child sees something that attracts him to the other side of the road, he may dash across, oblivious of the traffic. If he sees something on a high shelf, he will climb up to get it with complete disregard of house rules or safety. He may fall off furniture; if windows are left unguarded he may fall out. With any hyperactive child, doors and gates must be made secure; windows, fires and ovens guarded; gas-taps, water-taps, switches and power points covered and guarded and closely as possible, until a much later age than with the normal child.

The hyperactive child cannot remember instructions. A firm 'No' is forgotten within minutes, let alone days. Because his brain becomes intensely overstimulated by any mental exertion, instructions of any kind tend to evoke a wild and uncontrolled response. Telling a hyperactive five-year-old to put his vest on may just result in him rushing around the room, waving his vest wildly. Pressure may make him lie on the floor kicking and giggling. Anger will mean tears and tantrums, even fighting, biting or scratching, but it will not make him put his vest on!

If you can see it is a bad day (and days do vary) treat him as you would a much younger child and simply talk to him about other things to distract him while you dress him. Note what he had to eat the previous day, and accept that today he is not well enough to behave at a five-year-old level. This will make things easier for both of you. Trying to 'battle through' and 'make him see sense' while he is full of an allergic substance or toxin simply won't work, and the wear and tear on your nerves and his make it positively harmful.

Another problem area is sitting at the table. If you ask him to use a spoon or just to 'eat up' on a bad day, it may make him jump down and run round the table or disappear underneath it! Instead, simply pick up the spoon and feed him. Again note the previous meal and/or outside factors such as 'Is the gas fire on?', 'Has he been in the car?', 'Has he been exposed to cigarette smoke?' Remember, hyperactivity is an illness which affects behaviour and it is a problem with a solution. Try to blame the allergen or toxin, not the child.

Taking turns with other children is another difficult lesson. He may fight for first turn, the red counter, the mug with the picture on it, and to go on the slide again as soon as he reaches the bottom. Other children's rights must be respected and he *must* be restrained, but expect a violent reaction – it is typical of hyperactivity, not just of your child.

Be prepared to repeat many, many more times, all the edicts and instructions the normal child learns and remembers quite quickly.

Most hyperactive children do not respond to the voice alone. This is not deliberately ignoring the parent, but because they do not process incoming information in the normal way. Even the sound of their own name, repeated several times, may not get a response. Try touching the child to attract his attention. Get him to look at you and focus his attention on you before you speak. Shouting at him will produce more confusion in his brain and may make him run off or have a tantrum.

Running across the road, throwing stones at passing cars, dropping milk bottles or pot plants on passers-by from upstairs windows, putting ornaments down the lavatory, 'making waterfalls' by putting the plug in and turning on both taps in upstairs basins, climbing the garden gate and running off, getting up at 4 AM and taking the house apart, are the types of behaviour that *have* to be *effectively* prevented. Try to keep major rows to really important taboos, however.

If you have had a particularly noisy session, it is sometimes as well to explain to your neighbour what the problem was. Otherwise an extra-sympathetic smile and head-pat from the person next door (accompanied by a glare in the mother's direction) may undo all the good that the confrontation has just done!

The hyperactive child is very quick to pick up the nuances of 'poor little chap – his mother's very tough on him' which are frequently inspired by his rather appealing little face! But a hyperactive child whose confidence in his mother is undermined in this way has a double problem.

Be confident in how you are handling him, and share this confidence with your neighbours. Ask what *they* would do if *their* child got out of bed, climbed on the roof and started throwing stones down! Explain what you can – and then forget what they refuse to understand!

Sympathy from older people, who brought up families in an age before polluted crops, water, air and junk foods brought the problem of hyperactivity, may be scant at first. Enlightenment may come, however, as the child improves! 'I didn't believe a word of what you were telling me at first, but he is so much better since he came off additives, I'm beginning to think there must be something in it', is music to the ears of a hard-pressed parent!

Resist, however, the temptation to complain about him more than is necessary to explain specific situations – and always try to keep your attitude positive and constructive: 'He will be better in a few weeks when we have cleansed his lead out,' 'He's better in the summer, so we're having the gas boiler moved outside.' It is all too easy to be labelled 'that dreary mother with that ghastly little kid!'

While he is still very hyperactive it is best to avoid crowds and large gatherings where he is likely to be a pain to all present. If he cannot sit through prize-giving, a family wedding, the school play, or queue for the pleasure boats without fidgeting, grizzling or causing exasperation all round, it is as well to abandon such exercises for this year, or see if Granny will have him for the afternoon! Things will be better next year when the treatment has had time to take effect.

Some demands, however, must be made in the normal course of family life; when restraints necessarily arise, it is important to blame the *behaviour* and not the *child*, e.g. 'People don't do things like that' or 'That's a very naughty thing to do,' rather than 'You are a very naughty boy.' *He* is good; you and he are on the same side. *Bad temper, grabbing food, running away, hitting a friend* is naughty. *He*, being a good boy, mustn't do naughty things like that. You and he (the unit) don't do things like that. This message will take a long time to sink in, but in the end, you triumph together. He is your son and you love one another.

As the hyperactivity abates (and it may only take weeks to see a significant degree of improvement) more demands can be made. Point out how 'grown up' he is becoming and let his life become more complicated, a little at a time: 'You put on your socks and vest and I will help you with the rest;' 'You do three more spoonsful and then I will feed you.'

Tell other people how good and helpful he is being *in front* of him, and do not comment at all the days he backslides.

He will have to learn to do small household chores, to wait his turn with others, to *lose* at games and to develop skills requiring patience and dexterity. All of this is much harder for the hyperactive child than for the normal child, even after treatment, as he will have a big developmental backlog to make up. Maximum help should be given in the home, where his difficulties are understood, and all the family should remind him of chores, get him to put away toys, play games with him and *win* them, talk to him, help him accept it isn't his turn to choose the television programme, and generally give him as much 'life experience' as they can in his own home. Nowhere else will so much trouble be taken, so much understanding be shown, so much tolerance but firmness be exerted with even temper.

When he has improved noticeably, it is worth going to see his teacher, pointing out how much he has improved (and why!) and discussing his management with her. 'He will take turns now, if you are firm, and his speech is clearer. He will stop fidgeting if he is reminded, but we still need to touch his arm to get his attention when we speak to him ...' The more you can communicate with the school, the better the co-operation will be, but sometimes the attitudes are too entrenched to make this possible. Transferring to a school where the attitude is more sympathetic to hyperactivity may be a solution in some cases. Try to remember, though, when communicating with teachers and headmasters, what a pain he must be in a class of twenty! He may set other children off, or disturb or alienate them. Just imagine what having twenty of him would be like!

Playgroup and Nursery

In our experience it is important for parents to discuss their child's problems with the person running his Playgroup or Nursery class, with special reference to the child's food intolerance (if any) and chemical sensitivities (i.e. to food colourings, etc.) This is very important, as we have found that a number of young children do react to a number of items used, such as playdough, plasticine, finger paints, face paints, etc. We have known of cases where the child has broken out in rashes, and the cause has not been obvious.

The other likely problem is that drinks and biscuits, etc., are often provided which are not suitable for the hyperactive child. If your child is affected by his diet, it will be necessary to ask that he be allowed to take his own refreshments each day.

A quiet word will be all that is necessary, as we believe that more people are aware of additive and allergy problems now.

Primary school

Many hyperactive children suffer speech, hearing, vision and memory deficits and, coupled with their poor concentration, school becomes a frustrating and extremely difficult place for them.

For example, the 'open plan' type of classroom is extremely unsuitable for these children. They need a quiet and very structured curriculum if they are to make progress. They do well on a one-to-one basis.

For hyperactive children of pre-school and school age, additional educational support is very often needed, although difficult to obtain. All schools have a Special Educational Needs Co-ordinator (SENCO). Parents need to seek their help and advice. There are also a number of organisations which are able to support children with Special Education needs. Obtaining the help required, however, is not always an easy task. All Local Education Authorities (LEAs) have information available, and parents should contact their LEA for further assistance. *If your child is encountering difficulty at school it may help to give his teacher the fact sheet/ Teacher's Guide to Hyperactivity* (available from the HAC-SG; please send 65p in stamps to cover photocopying and postage fees).

Finally, what about the parents themselves? Being the parents of a hyperactive child must be one of the most exacting jobs the world has ever thrown up. You have to be constantly vigilant and aware of the danger he may be to himself and others, day and night. Your emotional responses, usually so finely-tuned to your own child, are constantly scrambled by the atypical responses of the hyperactive child. Being constantly on the receiving end of temper, or constantly apparently ignored, means your own reactions have to be exaggerated and emphasized every time you need to communicate, and with the hyperactive child, you have to communicate about once a minute.

But help is at hand. Parents of hyperactive children unite! Unite with each other and vow you are going to see your children back to normal in the next few years, come what may.

Unite with other parents who are lonely, harassed and confused, and isolated.

Unite with groups like HACSG who need help to spread the word. Write to Government ministers, headmasters, food manufacturers, school caterers, etc. Don't demand the impossible, but achieving things like custard-coloured custard (not pink!) should not be beyond us.

Unite with your children – follow their diet, it will help you too.

Ignore gossip and criticism (there may be lots) and try to educate all and sundry on the causes and care of hyperactive children.

TOMMY'S IMPROVEMENT CAUSES LEA TO REVIEW SCHOOL DINNER POLICY

THIS IS TOMMY'S STORY ...
    After many years' anguish resulting in my son Tommy's expulsion from his first school at the tender age of 7, I am happy to report that since being

on a wholesome, *additive-free* diet, his behaviour improved to such an extent that his new school teacher did not recognize him at the beginning of the new term!

The Head of Tommy's school was also equally astounded at the great improvement in his behaviour, and as a result agreed to arrange a meeting with the Local Education Authority's Head of Catering ... as Tommy had had a particularly bad incident after eating a school dinner.

The meeting was also attended by the catering company involved, as well as a Consultant Dietitian friendly to our cause.

I am pleased to say that as a result of this meeting the LEA have agreed to re-evaluate its school dinner policy, with particular reference to inclusion of any food additives, and will try to avoid their use whenever it is feasible.

In addition they say that they can always provide an individualized menu for any child with a special medical dietary requirement.

(With acknowledgement to HACSG, May 1997)

We need schools which are entirely aware of the problem of hyperactivity.

We need child-friendly wholefood lunches in the dining room, with filtered water or unadulterated fresh fruit juices.

Aluminium pans for cooking vegetables and/or fruit, additives, toxic chemicals such as cleaning materials, air-conditioning treatments and other items such as toxic felt-tip pens, need *removing*.

Vending machines selling foods that contribute to hyperactivity and ill-health should be replaced with school tuck shops selling healthy snacks and drinks.

In some schools there maybe big problems with children who come to school without breakfast. In some areas of the country 'breakfast clubs' have been set up and the teachers have said how much the children's behaviour and concentration have improved.

And it has recently been publicized that in one particular area local people have begun to 'dig for health' and are busy growing their own food. Children love 'growing things', they just need the encouragement and support of enthusiastic adults. Parents may like to get involved in raising funds to replace the fluorescent lighting and aluminium pans used in school, or for seeds or fruit bushes or even lending a hand to help the children 'dig for health.'

Lastly, it would enhance children's knowledge of nutrition and help to prepare them for later life, if cookery lessons making use of wholefood recipes were to be instated in the school curriculum.

CHAPTER 6

THE WAY FORWARD – PREVENTING HYPERACTIVITY

Many of you who read this book and do not have a hyperactive child of your own may wonder whether the effort involved in following the treatments we suggest is worth it. Few parents who have hyperactive children would. The day-to-day problems of coping with such a child are so much more arduous, the problems at school and fears for the future loom so large, that a little extra cooking and giving food supplements each day amount to nothing seen in the light of the child's improvement.

The beauty of the natural health approach we recommend is that it can do no harm – in fact it can do the whole family good. So often we hear how a younger brother's bed-wetting has stopped, or a mother's migraines have disappeared since the whole family have switched to the new diet.

The health and happiness of the family can start to spiral upwards instead of downwards as the diet helps the hyperactive child, and therefore the parents, tensions lessen, and the whole family benefits.

PREVENTION OF HYPERACTIVITY

Before conception

Can hyperactivity be prevented? We believe the answer is yes. The Foresight Association was formed in 1978 to combat disadvantage in child health by preparing men and women for parenthood by natural methods. It believes that:

1. Both parents should be on a good wholefood diet prior to conception.
2. Both parents should discontinue smoking well in advance of conception, as smoking in pregnancy correlates with hyperactivity in the baby after birth, premature birth, and deformity.
3. Both parents should avoid alcohol prior to conception (alcohol can damage sperm) and the mother for the duration of the pregnancy and during lactation, as alcohol squanders the B vitamins and some essential minerals. The deformities and mental retardation associated with foetal alcohol syndrome are now well-documented.
4. Women should come off the contraceptive pill at least six months before the intended pregnancy and use a barrier method of contraception instead. (The Pill squanders zinc, magnesium and B complex vitamins.)
5. The couple should try to make sure they are free from infections, including genito-urinary infections, or intestinal parasites, heavy metal toxicities and trace mineral deficiencies well in advance of pregnancy. (There are now a number of clinics where Foresight consultants can give advice on this.)
6. As a very high percentage of hyperactive children are born into allergic families, and very many have mothers who suffer from migraine (which is often due to food allergy), it is extremely important food allergies are

checked, if possible before conception. Babies can be sensitized to cow's milk intolerance in the womb, and if mothers are unaware of these possibilities, infants can suffer a cascade of health and behavioural problems.

7. Hair analyses to detect mineral deficiencies and toxicities, and a nutritional programme to correct these, can be obtained from Foresight (see Useful Addresses).

By taking these precautions and avoiding toxic and allergenic substances prior to conception, we believe we can substantially increase the chances of the pregnancy starting well.

Pregnancy and birth

Dietary precautions and avoidance of toxic and allergenic substances should continue throughout the pregnancy.

The birth itself should be as natural and drug-free as possible (a very high percentage of births can be totally drug-free) followed by demand-feeding of colostrum and breast-milk.

Breast-milk and particularly colostrum, the milk secreted by the human breast during the first days after the birth, is rich in substances that confer immunity on the baby when he is most susceptible to life-threatening infections. Breast-milk is rich in antibodies. These proteins are necessary for the body's defence against infection by bacteria and viruses.

Breast-feeding

In most cases, the demand-fed baby will feed very frequently for the first four to six days – a little and often is the best way to prepare and develop the immature digestive tract. After the first week, times between feeds should increase as the mother's milk becomes more plentiful.

For the mother a good varied diet, rich in unsaturated fats and vitamins and minerals, is the best way to promote a sufficient supply of good quality milk. Talk about 'resting' and 'relaxing' is all very fine, but except in the case of the first baby, it is seldom possible! Fear of being unable to relax as often as the experts prescribe may inhibit milk flow; as may assurances that 'if you worry your milk will go.' If the milk supply is going, it is due to insufficient nutrients – that is *why* the mother is worrying! If she eats well, takes vitamin and mineral supplements, puts the baby to the breast when he cries, the milk will flow in.

Where the mother is taking a good diet and sensible supplementation, separate vitamin supplements for the baby should not be necessary. Her breast-milk should be of sufficiently good quality to alleviate the need to give the baby fish-liver oils, rosehip syrup, etc. Giving breast-milk alone often prevents the early allergic syndromes. Some breast-fed babies have attacks of colic (crying and pulling up their legs) if the mother is drinking cow's milk. Some studies have shown that they are much more settled if their mother gives up drinking cow's milk and avoids cow products in general. This is well worth trying if the child is unsettled. Water is the best drink for nursing mothers.

Mixed feeding

With breast-feeding going well, mixed feeding can probably be postponed until about seventeen to twenty weeks – except in the case of the unusually large and hearty baby, who may be ready for solids from about fifteen weeks.

The first tastes should be of very finely sieved foods, just a teaspoonful in the first instance. Only one new food should be given on each day, and if the food appears not to suit him, it should be *discontinued immediately* and not reintroduced for some months.

Little helpings should be worked up a teaspoonful at a time; the child should not be pressed to eat more than he needs. Very small amounts at two or three feeds will be better than one large meal. By six months, he may be taking a little baby rice at breakfast, with a teaspoonful of egg yolk (hard-boiled and sieved); a few teaspoonsful of bone broth with sieved vegetables for lunch; a few teaspoonsful of sieved fruit for tea, followed each time by a plentiful breast-feed. Quantities should be very gradually increased as his enthusiasm for the food grows.

Different cereals can be introduced for breakfast, with a little helping of fruit or a drink of fruit juice, with egg yolk (hard-boiled and sieved) on alternate days. At lunch time, herring roes or pounded chicken, liver or fish, can be added to the strained vegetables and broth. Until at least eight months, breast-milk will remain the optimal second course. At supper time, rusk soaked in milk or milk pudding can be given with mashed banana or sieved fruit, raw or stewed. Very gradually, a little at a time, items from the family meal can be added in, mashed, sieved or blended.

Once he is about nine to twelve months old, he will be able to sit happily in a high chair and join in family meals.

Lumpy food should not be given to the child before he is ready to chew it up. Giving him adult foods a few months too soon, so that large lumps of indigestible substances arrive in his stomach and cause acidity and colic, is a frequent source of night screaming, skin rashes, irritability, diarrhoea and other allergic syndromes. He may not become a dab hand at chewing until he has cut the molars that come through at about 18 months, and many children need their meat shredded up very finely until they have cut their two-year-old molars.

Feeding fresh, finely sieved or mashed foods, in very small amounts at first, while continuing to breast-feed four to five times a day, is the best way to avoid setting up any adverse reaction – be it allergy, intolerance or sensitivity.

If a food 'does not suit him' – i.e., produces crying (pain), diarrhoea, nappy rash, other skin rashes, weeping cradle-cap, running nose, wheezing, coughing or other adverse symptoms, this should *not* be ignored. He is not having a 'temper tantrum', it is not 'just one of those things', he is having an allergic reaction. *The warning signs should not be ignored.* Keeping a diet diary can be helpful (see page 51).

Colic is another sign that the infant may be suffering from a food intolerance. It is important that parents seek help from their GP to have this checked (see page 50).

To keep pushing a food into a child if it does not suit him, not only makes for an unhappy, grizzly baby, it may make for a sickly, hyperactive child for years to come. Letting him thrive on foods that suit him will help him to build up a good constitution, and later he may well be able to tolerate a wide variety of foods.

A sleepless night with a child when he is not actively teething or suffering from an infection needs investigation. What did he eat the previous day? The answer should be written down – if necessary even at two in the morning! – so it can be checked if it recurs. This way allergies can be spotted and eliminated right from the outset and many sleepless nights avoided for all the family.

If despite all efforts sleep patterns are poor, and appetite and temperament unreliable, it may be worth having a hair analysis as soon as he has enough hair. Meanwhile bottled or filtered water may help, as may avoiding areas of crowded traffic. The child should be kept away from cigarette smoke, and his meals should not be prepared in aluminium saucepans.

These are some of the practical, day-to-day ways we may be able to avoid hyperactivity in our children. On a more long-term basis we can join – or form – groups which are trying to eliminate some of the dangers from our environment, be it lead in petrol or colouring in food.

But above all we need to spread the word – books in the recommended reading list will give an insight into the work we are doing. It is only fair to the next generation of children that we spread this knowledge before they are conceived – we could make the families, schools, and above all the *children* of the future so much happier.

SO WHERE ARE WE AT?

Some of you may have read the first edition of this book, published in 1984, and you may well be wondering why there has been so little progress with public awareness or medical knowledge of how to help these children in the intervening 14 years. Indeed, in view of the widespread havoc in schools, the 'unemployability' of so many learning disabled young, and the increase in drug-taking and crime, it is strange that so little attention has been paid to this whole area. If we are to make progress, we must try to understand why this is so. To start with, why is so much ridicule levelled at two very straightforward theories?

First, the theory that food colourings and other additives, pollutants (as well as some commonly eaten foods, which are ingested in large quantities) can affect brain cells, and thus have an adverse effect on mood and behaviour. As we have explained in this book, numbers of research scientists have reported a range of adverse reactions, including eczema, asthma, migraine, epilepsy – and even hyperactivity! This research has been published, much of it in the 1960s and 1970s.

Nobody would argue that alcohol, antidepressants, tranquillizers, sleeping pills, painkillers, anaesthetics and street drugs do not affect the brain and alter reactions. Why then are organizations such as HACSG ridiculed for saying food colourings affect children, when the very people who scoff are then putting the children onto medication. Is there any logic here?

Secondly, why is the knowledge rejected that nutrients such as calcium, magnesium, zinc, manganese, B complex vitamins and so on can affect health, growth, vitality, brain development and mood and behaviour *positively*? If we look again at all the books and papers on nutrition the facts are there. The word 'hyperactivity' crops up time and again as effects of nutrient deficiencies are described in deprived animals. Rats, pigs, rabbits, mice and monkeys are studied, and hyperactivity is noted.

Why do doctors not study the available research? Are we, the taxpayers, funding medical research purely for the benefit of future rat populations? Or can it be that the work is for the benefit of the scientists only? Once money has been paid for a study, can it be put on a shelf somewhere, while funding for another study is negotiated and carried through? Many pharmaceutical companies fund the research in universities. Are these studies carried out just so that the next childhood plague can be forecast, so huge mountains of the appropriate medicaments can be stockpiled?

Be that as it may, the research *is* available if searched for, in some very useful books, listed at the end of this book. Many parents and carers may like not only to read these, but also to lend them to their doctors and health visitors, and the head teacher of their child's school.

It seems it is up to parents to take the lead. It seems this has not been well understood in the past. Now the time has come. Join the HACSG. Make waves. Make changes.

CHAPTER 7

SPECIAL DIETS

The following diets have been used by parents of hyperactive children and found to be helpful.

THE FEINGOLD FOOD PROGRAMME

This food programme was devised by the late Dr Ben Feingold in the US. On p.98 we give excerpts from letters we have had from parents who have used it with their hyperactive children in this country.

The background

Quoted from 'Food additives, the Feingold Diet and Hyper-activity.'

Elimination diets and specific testing suggest that food additives may be a factor in many cases of childhood hyperactivity. Dr Ben F. Feingold of Kaiser-Permanente Medical Center has reduced hyperactivity in children by placing them on a diet free of salicylates, artificial flavours and colours. Dr Feingold investigated adverse reactions to drugs and food additives, all low-molecular weight compounds. He found that aspirin (acetylsalicylic acid) and the salicylates in foods and some synthetic flavours cause allergic reactions in sensitive people. When other researchers reported that the commonly-used food dye tartrazine (UK E102;FD and C yellow 5 in the US) caused reactions in aspirin–sensitive patients, Feingold designed a diet free of all artificial flavours and colours, aspirin, and natural salicylates. The diet was initially prescribed for patients with itching, hives, skin rashes, anxiety and asthma. When these allergic reactions and also the mental symptoms improved, Feingold began using the diet to treat hyperactive children! Fifty per cent of the children put on the diet responded fully, while 70 per cent improved enough to be taken off drugs.

Since the first edition of this book was published in 1984, there have been a large number of controlled research studies, from countries worldwide, which support Dr Feingold's hypothesis. It has also been shown through research by Dr G. Kroyer of the Institute of Technology, University of Vienna, that food colourings can inhibit certain important digestive enzymes. In addition, Dr Kroyer found that some food colours destroy vitamin C in processed foods within four days.

In 1995, 1996 and 1997 the HACSG had several meetings (at their invitation) with officials from the Ministry of Agriculture Fisheries and Food, and the Department of Health. The authors of this book were asked to give a forty-minute presentation regarding our work, and latest research, to the

Committee on Toxicity of Chemicals in Food, Consumer Products and the Environment (COT). COT were very impressed by this presentation, and a Working Party has been set up to make a very full study of food intolerance and reactions to food additives. We look forward to the results. Many of the so-called 'research studies' which have been carried out with reference to the Feingold Diet have seriously misrepresented Dr Feingold's hypothesis, and *none* of the studies rigidly followed the strict guidelines which he had laid down.

It must also be remembered that we are now in the second (sometimes third) generation of children whose parents have had a diet containing many artificial additives, plus quite serious pollution of the environment. As one of our medical advisers says, these children are the *first* 'food additive and antibiotic generation'.

How does the Feingold Diet correlate with the high lead, copper and low zinc findings?
Salicylates, benzoates, and tartrazine and chelating agents will 'grab onto' the essential trace elements and interfere with their absorption. Of the three, the most active is probably the yellow dye tartrazine; the least active is the benzoate molecule. The intestinal contents contain partially-digested food with various concentrations of copper, zinc, iron, lead, calcium and magnesium. Grains contain phytate, which decreases the absorption of zinc because phytate is a known chelating agent. These chelating agents are more specific for some metals than for others. Therefore the absorption of copper and lead could be increased by salicylates and tartrazine, while the absorption of zinc could be decreased. Orotic acid in milk whey is also a

chelating agent and therefore may be a factor in hyperactivity. These additives could thereby increase hyperactivity in children who have a high level of lead and copper in their food and drink and a low level of zinc and calcium. This is a testable hypothesis which would take much of the mystery out of the food allergy story.

Since salicylates and food additives evidently do enhance some types of hyperactivity, placing a child on the Feingold Diet might relieve the condition and certainly would do no harm. The mode of action of the dyes and salicylates may be owing to the chemical chelating effect which these compounds have on trace elements.

How to begin

1. Read with care everything you can on the Feingold food programme, including Dr Feingold's book *Why Your Child is Hyperactive* (see Recommended Reading).
2. Keep a diet diary, noting everything the individual eats and drinks, along with a side-by-side record of behaviour and sleep patterns, so that these can be compared. This record should be kept even after success with the programme is achieved. In the event of an unfavourable reaction, the diet record makes it easy to determine which food caused the problem.
3. The greatest success is observed when the entire family adheres to the programme. This requires the commitment and support of all family members. When the prohibited foods are not present in the house, temptation and the risk of infractions are reduced. The all-out effort by all family members serves as an added incentive to the child. Many families have found that the elimination of

the non-essential additives often benefits other members of the family as well, both children and adults.

4. This food programme must be adhered to 100 per cent. Compliance of 90 per cent does not yield a 90 per cent improvement, but rather leads to disappointment. A single bite or sip can lead to a reaction that may last for 72 hours.

5. Reading food labels is very important. However, you should realize that some labels can be misleading and regulations are far too many to quote individually here. It is best not to buy anything which says it contains 'preservatives', 'colour' or 'flavouring' though 'natural colouring' and 'natural flavouring' should be all right.

6. The key is to be selective at the supermarket. Once the food is in the house it is too late to determine if it is 'safe'. It is hard to tell a child 'no' to something he already has in his hands.

7. Please let bakers, butchers and food manufacturers know that you want pure non-additive foods for your family. When asking about food, it is not enough to say 'Is it all natural?' You will get a more helpful response if you are specific: 'Is it made with real or imitation vanilla? Are there any preservatives in it?' etc.

8. *Away from home* As it is very important that your child adheres to the diet, it is advisable to send a packed lunch for school. If the headteacher will not agree, please let the HACSG know. Your doctor or health visitor may help here. Most headteachers are very cooperative once they understand the situation. If your child is bothered by refusing 'treats' when away from home, suggest this response: 'Thank you, but I am sensitive to artificial colours and flavours.' Some children find it easier to say 'I'm allergic' (although this sensitivity is not allergy according to the medical definition of allergy). Usually this approach will elicit a sympathetic response on the

part of his friends, whereas 'I'm on a diet' may prompt ridicule. When there is a birthday party most hostesses will not be insulted if you telephone ahead and explain the difficulty, ask what is on the menu and send substitutions. In time he may report back that the mother of the birthday-child is going to join the 'programme' because so many brought their own food and drink!

9. *Medicines* When drugs have been prescribed a physician should be notified before making any changes in the medication. Since many drugs are synthetically coloured and flavoured, ask your physician or pharmacist to prescribe non-coloured/flavoured drugs and medicines. Behaviour-modifying drugs, aside from containing colour and flavouring, have been known to have long-lasting residual effects. If your child has been on these drugs, it may be necessary to wait longer to see the desired effect of the diet.

General comments taken from responses to the HACSG's questionnaire on the Feingold food programme

It's like living with a different child, one I always thought was 'in there', but trapped by his excruciating behaviour! He can now concentrate, tie laces, dress himself, does not scream anymore, can participate in sports. (He was extremely disruptive at school and very destructive at home.)

M seems to have undergone a complete change (noticeable after one to two months of diet). She is very careful what she eats because reactions have caused her some distress. We are all much happier.

What a relief from the day-to-day hassle. At last a full night's sleep. T is a different child in more ways than one. I am also fully weaned off tranquillizers thanks to the Feingold diet.

Have found L greatly improved. Sometimes has bad days but generally is a much happier, calmer and better behaved child and is definitely less aggressive and has fewer temper tantrums.

Thank you so much. Our life is a life now instead of a living hell. No one can understand unless they have been there!

Lapses in diet result in such drastic relapses in behaviour that sceptical relatives and friends have become convinced. Have successfully recommended diet to other parents.

Everyone we know, and school, say how much better T is. A changed child!

Child has improved beyond recognition. This time last year we had an 'unteachable' daughter according to infant school and we were worried about how she would cope in the Juniors. But, since going on the diet she is managing just great!

Calmer child makes life both inside and outside the house more pleasant for all. Friends have commented how much calmer S is.

C is now a normal happy child on the diet and if given food he is 'allergic' to, the reaction is noticeable to anyone.

Child growing tall and well – healthy and bright-eyed.

Family life is less fraught now ...

Child much improved – discharged from doctor and I have had no more of the chest infections I used to have.

Our lives have completely changed since the diet – it was like a nightmare before.

The atmosphere in our home is now more relaxed.

I firmly believe the diet has worked for my son, I only wish I had used it sooner.

The diet has helped immensely, but I think that a lot of the problems developed because of his being hyperactive so long, these will take some time to sort out, but this is now possible because he is much calmer and more cooperative (boy aged 8 years).

Whole family on the diet – other children are much healthier too.

We are healthier and more relaxed as a result of the diet and we consequently enjoy life more and achieve more.

I wish the medical profession would take more notice of it.

All have better health and tempers.

Health of whole family improved – sinusitis, eczema, mouth ulcers have gone.

General improvement in health and growth but greatest improvement in temperament after giving vitamin B.

Child has not needed any *drugs* since the diet took effect after three to four weeks.

Without the diet I think we would have all gone round the bend.

Surprised at the amount of food additives, colouring, etc. in today's food.

This list could be repeated over and over again.

Extracts from letters from parents of hyperactive children who have been using the Feingold Food Programme.

Since reading your article we have dropped all monosodium glutamate from his diet and all fruit juices and in three weeks we can see an improvement – we have had two nights of undisturbed sleep and to me and my husband that is heaven – also his general outlook is better – he doesn't cry all the time and his nightmares and sleepwalking are much better.

(Baby 14 months old)

Before she was put on the diet she was very excitable and overactive; she had many tantrums, often one or two a day and had excessive crying sessions. She was unhappy and very bad tempered, her power of concentration was poor and her speech was bad, very muddled – she has to attend speech therapy. Since starting the diet there have been vast improvements. Gone are the daily tantrums and excessive crying bouts. She has definitely slowed down to a much more normal pace and her speech has started to improve rapidly ... she is now most definitely a much happier little girl. And my husband and myself and family are absolutely thrilled with the most outstanding results to date.

(Girl aged 5)

I have now had baby on the diet for just over two weeks. Even friends who don't see him often have commented on the difference, so I really believe this is what has been the trouble. After crying tears of relief and remorse for all the times I've screamed 'for God's sake shut up' I am now taking a real joy and pride in my lovely son instead of loving him with gritted teeth ... Last week he *actually slept* on three separate days till 5.30–6 AM and settled again after a drink. His concentration has improved a thousandfold ... I am so enthusiastic over this I would help anyone.

(Boy 1 year old)

'A totally different child' ... We found the Headmistress hard going at first, but she changed her tune when D started his diet and took a packed lunch, because the change has been UNBELIEVABLE!!!

We found the diet worked almost immediately. At first we had a lot of problems at school, and only now am I feeling more happy about the situation. I only wished we had put him on the diet earlier. I feel cheated that we've missed out so much, because of all the rubbish in foods. We find the older generation find it hard to accept about E numbers. Many thanks.

(Boy aged 7)

Eight months ago I put my son on the diet. We now have a healthy, contented child who I have not had to take to the doctors for 6 months. It used to be six weeks. I would be more than willing to give any assistance if required to the local contact.

(Boy aged 5)

THE 'CAVEMAN' DIET

This diet was devised by Dr Elizabeth Lodge-Rees of California. It is essentially an 'elimination' diet which is used first to identify foods which may produce a bad reaction and then to rebuild a healthy diet. The name 'Caveman' emphasizes the need to eliminate modern processed foods. The basic principles are:

1. Determine which foods we use today would have been used before frozen or processed foods.
2. Accept that the bad effects of previous diet may take four to five weeks to be eliminated from the body.
3. Sugar and flour-based products are *out* (i.e., sweets, ice cream, biscuits, cakes, puddings).
4. Most cereal-based foods are *out* (i.e., white flour, breakfast cereals, including cornflakes, rice) unless they are complete, i.e., wholemeal flour, brown rice, possibly oatmeal (although with some children these may still be suspect).

5. Milk and dairy foods (butter, cream, cheese) are also suspect – as is margarine.
6. Added salt should only be rock or sea-salt, as proprietary brands frequently have supplements or additives to make them free-running.
7. Only *water* should be drunk – *no* tea, coffee, chocolate, cola drinks, diet drinks, or malted drinks, milk or squash.

SUGGESTIONS FOR A GLUTEN-FREE, MILK-FREE, EGG-FREE DIET

Try to vary the dishes every day.

Breakfast

Bacon with kidney, liver, mushrooms, tomatoes**, bananas, prunes**, apple rings**, or sautéed potatoes.

Fish: plain baked or grilled; kedgeree can be made with rice and sweetcorn, from smoked haddock, smoked mackerel or sardines; tuna, sardines or smoked mackerel can be eaten cold with bean shoots.

Raw fruit** and fruit juices**.

Goats' or soy milk, if tolerated. Milkshakes made with banana or any soft fruit** and honey. Also nice with cashew butter, or just plain honey.

Lunch

Any fresh meat, fish, poultry or offal, with two or three vegetables, potato or rice. Gravies or sauces must be thickened with arrowroot, cornflour or split-pea flour.

Raw or stewed fruit**. If goats' or soy milk is tolerated, puddings can be made with plain, flaked or ground rice, sago, cornflour or gluten-free semolina (obtainable from Boots).

Supper

Soups
Bone broth made from bone jelly. Thicken with peas, beans, lentils, split-pea flour or potato. Add meat scraps and vegetables such as carrots, leeks, onions, mushrooms, swedes, beets, etc.

Salads
Any raw fruit** and vegetable such as lettuce, endive, cucumber, apple, date, beet, carrot, tomato, coleslaw, cress, sprouted seeds, etc. Dressing made with safflower oil, cider vinegar** and honey. Baked or boiled potato. Sardine, tuna, cold meats, prawns, cold fish, etc. Most meat and fish pastes (check the label).

Puddings
Goat or soy milkshake. Juice.

Dried fruits**: sultanas, raisins, pears, apricots, peaches.
Nuts: walnuts, almonds, brazils, cashews.

Rice cakes with honey; jam**, *Marmite*, cashew nut butter.

THE HYPERACTIVE CHILDREN'S SUPPORT GROUP

The Hyperactive Children's Support Group was founded in November 1977 and grew into a national association almost overnight. It was accorded charitable status in May 1979.

The aims of the Group are 'to help and support hyperactive children and their parents; to conduct research and promote investigation into the incidence of hyperactivity in the UK – its causes and treatments; and to disseminate information concerning this condition'. The condition itself goes by a few names: Attention Deficit Disorder (AD), Hyperactive Disorder (HD) and Hyperactivity (HA).

Many children are hyperactive from birth (they are often HA in utero); they are restless, fidgety, sleep perhaps three to four hours out of 24 and cry almost incessantly. They will not feed properly, whether breast or bottle fed, and may also suffer from asthma and eczema. The mother is completely bewildered by this, especially if it is her first baby – no amount of nursing, cuddling, or comforting will pacify such a child.

As these children grow older this hyperactive behaviour is accentuated – they seem in a state of perpetual motion, which makes them extremely accident prone. Although a high IQ is possible, many HA children experience difficulty in learning;

speech can be a problem, and often balance is poor, with extreme clumsiness. They are prone to cot-rocking and head banging; their behaviour is unpredictable and disruptive; they are easily excitable and cry often; they are unable to sit still for more than a few minutes at a time; coordination and concentration are very poor. They are poor sleepers and eaters. There is often a history of headaches, ear infections, catarrh, asthma, hay fever, and other respiratory complaints; and boys are more likely to be affected than girls. Another strange symptom which has emerged from many letters from parents is that almost all HA children suffer from abnormal thirst.

We believe that a connection may exist between baby battering and hyperactivity, since in many cases the condition is not diagnosed and most parents have never heard of hyperactivity.

Parents have written to say that they feel 'loners' and social outcasts. They feel their children create such havoc wherever they go that they are not welcome in playgroups, nursery school, shops, friends' or relatives' homes. A simple shopping trip takes on nightmarish qualities.

Many of these babies and children are prescribed a succession of drugs to try and control this behaviour, but even in adult dosage, drugs give poor results.

SALLY BUNDAY TELLS HER OWN STORY

My own son Miles was born hyperactive and for six long years we battled with his exhausting behaviour; the only treatment offered was a succession of drugs, none of which seemed very effective. Then quite by chance I heard about a diet which Dr Ben Feingold (Chief Emeritus, Department of Allergy, Kaiser Permanents Medical Center, San Francisco) had formulated from his researches as an allergist. I lost no time in sending for this and after *four days* of starting Miles on it he was a changed child – he actually slept the night, which in itself was a small miracle.

The diet is a very simple one. It is designed to eliminate as far as possible synthetic chemical additives from a person's diet, i.e. colours, flavours, MSG, BHA, BHT and others; and for the first four to six weeks only certain fruits and vegetables which contain natural salicylates; salicylates are 'aspirin like' chemicals to which HA children are often sensitive. Gradually the suspect fruits can be reintroduced and if no adverse response is noted they can be added to the daily menus.

Miles responded well to the diet; he became much calmer and was able to sit at the table to eat a proper meal; he learnt to read quite quickly, was much less disruptive at school, and altogether he is a much happier little boy.

My health visitor was so astounded at the change in Miles that she recommended the diet to other mothers who were experiencing difficulties with their children: before long it was obvious that I would not be able to cope single-handed with all the enquiries which came pouring in and several kind friends helped me form the Group.

I adapted the Feingold Food Programme for British foods.

We at the HACSG publish a handbook, *Hyperactive children: A guide to their management*, which includes full details of the Feingold Programme, listing foods 'allowed' and 'not allowed', and complete information on those fruits/vegetables which contain naturally occurring salicylates. The booklet includes 'Ideas for meals' which we think helps parents when first beginning the programme. The booklet also contains ideas for management, educational problems, avoidance of stress for the child, together with a checklist on relevant research studies, including the HACSG study on Essential Fatty Acids.

Membership is on an annual basis, with three journals to keep members up-to-date on the latest information which comes to us from various sources, items on research, recipes, additions to the 'safe' foods guide, etc.

The diet is really a very healthy one, and most parents find it easier to keep the whole family on it, rather than having 'different' food in the house. Any infraction of the diet by the child may have serious consequences, with a reversion to behaviour disturbances.

In the first five years we had 40,000 requests for help. Since then countless thousands of distraught parents have written or telephoned for our information, advice and practical help. We are pleased to say that very many HA children have shown good improvements in health, behaviour and also learning, so that they have been better able to cope in school and within the family.

LOCAL GROUPS

We have a number of local parent contacts throughout the UK. These are proving extremely helpful and supportive, as new members are able to share experiences and make new friends who understand and sympathize. New members are put in touch with their local contact when they join the HACSG.

Parents are finding that with the lifting of their burden of guilt (they are often accused of being the cause of their child's hyperactivity, that they have mismanaged the child, etc.), they have much more confidence in themselves; with happier parents and a calmer child, families are really beginning to enjoy being a family.

We are also in correspondence with hyperactive support groups in Australia, New Zealand, Canada and the US.

OTHER CAUSES

There are other causes of HA, such as hypoglycaemia, milk allergy, food allergies, nutritional deficiency and possibly environmental pollution. However, we feel that the Feingold diet is something which parents may try for themselves; it contains no drugs, is based on simple fresh foods, and is entirely beneficial. Our advice to parents is to try the diet for two to three months and if you need help we can advise further.

Ideally, of course, every HA child should have a thorough examination and specialist diagnosis so that the causes can be pinpointed; however, until this disability is widely understood, this is not always possible.

RESEARCH

An important aim is research. It is not known for certain how many hyperactive (AD/HD) children and adolescents there are in the UK. The HACSG hopes to be able to help with this research.

In 1979 a number of children were tested at Aston University to see if they had an overload of toxic metals such as lead. This was not found, but what the research showed was that many of the children, and especially the boys, had a deficiency of zinc. Some were very deficient in this essential trace element. Since then many children belonging to the HACSG have been tested, and almost all have been found to be zinc-deficient. Zinc is especially important for the immune system, and the brain.

HACSG were the first to discover that these children were 'abnormally thirsty'. This is cardinal sign of a lack of Essential Fatty Acids. Our research hypothesis 'A Lack of Essential Fatty Acids as a Cause of Hyperactivity in Children', was based on the questionnaires and studies we had done with families in the HACSG (see page 115).

In 1995 and in 1996 at the prestigious Purdue University in the US, studies were published which showed that hyperactive children (AD/HD children) were deficient in these Essential Fatty Acids, which completely vindicated our work of 1981; work which had been ignored by most of the professionals, and indeed the Government.

In 1987 700+ families completed a long questionnaire, and this has been used as the basis of our database housed at the University of Surrey (under Dr Neil Ward, Senior Lecturer in Analytical Chemistry). Full details of the results are available, for a nominal sum, from HACSG (see also p. 110).

HACSG has also co-operated in a research study into a possible deficiency of vitamin B_{12} in some HA children. A pilot study showed that these children had a very high combination of factors, any one of which would cause B_{12} deficiency. The research is continuing at the Royal Free Hospital, by the Children's Medical Charity.

As a charity we at the HACSG continue to endeavour to raise funds for further research into this soul-destroying disability.

We are anxious to keep in touch with as many members of the medical profession, educationalists, etc. as possible; every scrap of information and feedback is essential in the research.

Colourings
Colourings are no longer permitted in foods described, either directly or by implication, as being especially prepared for infants and young children (except natural colours E101, E101a and E160a). The Government Food Additives and Contaminants Committee has recommended the following bans:

Nitrites and Nitrates
Legislation (similar to above conditions) enacted in 'Preservatives in Food Regulations' Amendment No. 15, February 1982.

Flavour Modifiers
Legislation (similar to above) enacted in Miscellaneous Additives in Food Regulations No. 14, 1983.

PREGNANCY

We would ask that special help and advice be given to mothers-to-be so that they understand the *great importance* of good nutrition for themselves and their baby from the beginning of pregnancy. We urge avoidance of foods containing the previously mentioned chemical additives, both in pregnancy and when breast-feeding. Also, if mothers suspect that they may suffer from a food intolerance (one indication is migraine), then they should ask to have tests carried out. The HACSG can provide information on migraine 'trigger' foods.

VULNERABILITY OF VERY YOUNG INFANTS

(WHO Food Additives Report 1971. Page 33, para. 4.1.) Very young infants are especially vulnerable to foreign chemicals because the mechanisms that provide protection against these substances are absent or not fully developed. Although the evidence for this derives mainly from studies with drugs rather than with food additives, it is likely that such very young infants are less efficient than older children in metabolizing some food additives and may therefore accumulate them to excessive levels. If this occurs at a time when sensitivity to toxic effects is critical because of the delicately balanced growth and differentiation processes, there may be deleterious consequences that may not appear until much later in the child's development. Very young infants may also differ from older children in relation to physiological barriers protecting sensitive tissues, such as the blood brain barrier or the protective barriers for retinal or lens (eye) tissue.

CONCLUSION

All we ask for is open minds on the subject of the dietary approach to this multiple disability. We are pleased to report that many doctors are considering this as an alternative to drug therapy, especially when they have seen for themselves the results in previously intransigent hyperactivity.

We have letters from parents saying that cases of severe migraine, asthma, eczema, epilepsy, dyslexia, and recently a case of severe mental disability, have responded to the nutritional approach.

INFORMATION ABOUT THE HACSG

Free information about the group, including our initial leaflet, is available from HACSG, 71 Whyke Lane, Chichester, West Sussex, PO19 2LD (an S.A.E. is very much appreciated).

Membership is on an annual basis, and parents on benefit are entitled to lower fees. Renewal fees are lower for all members.

A free copy of our handbook 'Hyperactive Children, A guide to their management' is sent to each member.

Members are entitled to three free journals per year, information about local Contacts in their area, free advice and help (as far as we are able), as well as to access to research and other information.

Our Handbook may be purchased separately and (as at May 1997) costs £3.50 (including p & p). (If a copy of the Handbook only is required, please send cheque or postal order for £3.50, and mark your envelope 'HANDBOOK ONLY PLEASE'. This will speed up despatch.) This includes full details of the Feingold Food Programme, list of food additives to avoid (including E numbers), list of local Contacts, Articles and reprints list, and 'Shopping Basket' guide. The Handbook also has a lot of information on allergies, stress, schooling and many other items to help parents.

See page 117 for a copy of the Group's General Information Sheet.

FINANCIAL HELP

Disability living allowance, attendance and mobility allowances are available. D.L.A. is in two parts, 'Help with getting around' and 'Help with personal care'. Children (getting around) is only applicable for children of five or over.

'Help with personal care' is available for babies and children of any age, *but they must need more help than children of the same age, and must have needed help for three months.*

Form D.I.A. 1 is available from Social Security offices, libraries and post offices. The Freephone number for enquiries is 0800 882 200.

In a letter to the HACSG the Department of Health says that 'Under certain circumstances it is possible for families on low incomes to obtain financial assistance from the DSS. Parents on low incomes can apply for Income Support from the DSS Benefits Agency by telling them of the "special dietary needs" of their child/children at the time of applying for benefit.'

The Rowntree Family Fund offers help in both cash and kind for especially difficult problems. Please write to Sally Bunday c/o the HACSG for an application form. The fund is very kind and helpful, so don't hesitate to ask. Items they have given include washing machines and freezers, if these would ease the problem of looking after a particularly difficult child. Children do have to be severely hyperactive to qualify for help.

The Medic Alert Foundation, 12 Bridge Wharf, 156 Caledonian Road, London, N1 9UU (Tel. 0171 833 3034) will send you information on bracelets or necklets which can be engraved to show if your child has a specific 'allergy' or asthma, epilepsy, or similar problems, or if he reacts violently to coloured drugs, chemicals, etc. These are not cheap, but would be helpful if your child spends some time away from home. Your GP's signature is required on the form.

HACSG DATABASE

The HACSG Database is housed at the Department of Chemistry, University of Surrey, and supervised by our Research Director, Dr Neil Ward.

DATABASE QUESTIONNAIRE 1987

357 Diagnosed Hyperactive Children (mixed ages) reacted to the following (highest %):

Synthetic colours	89%
Synthetic flavours	72%
Preservatives	72%
Antioxidants	50%
Monosodium Glutamate	60%
All synthetic additives	45%
Cow's milk & dairy	50%
Chocolate	60%
Orange	48%

Percentage of families with health problems

Migraine	65%
Asthma	52%
Eczema	51%
Hayfever	60%
Arthritis	55%
Food Allergies	60%
Chemical Allergies	40%

357 Diagnosed Hyperactive Children (*babies/infants only*)

Active *in utero*	72%
Crying & screaming	73%
Restless	85%
Woke in night	60%
Colicky	69%
Poor appetite	50%
Head banging	45%
Excessive dribbling	53%
Very very thirsty	75%
Prescribed antibiotics	70%
Prescribed sleeping drugs	40%

Slightly Older Children: 5–11 years. Percentage with problems. Symptoms improved on Feingold diet only. *No nutritional supplements given.*

Clumsiness	75%
Aggression	80%
Impulsiveness	90%
Poor coordination	60%
Seems unnaturally strong	75%
Learning difficulties	55%
Excessively argumentative	60%
Aggressive to parents/siblings	35%

357 Diagnosed Hyperactive Children Health & Behaviour problems. Overall 87% responded to Feingold Diet. *No nutritional supplements given.*

Allergic to foods	60%
Chemicals	40%
Eczema	42%
Diarrhoea	50%
Ear infections	58%
Chest infections	50%
Rashes	53%
Catarrh	60%
Night sweats	45%
Gut problems	42%

The next Database will be published early in 1998.

HACSG RESEARCH PAPER

The HACSG's research paper, 'A Lack of Essential Fatty Acids as a possible cause of Hyperactivity in Children', was based on the following findings.

The results of an HACSG Survey showed that

1. Seventy-four (74%) of boys and 75% of girls showed good response to the Feingold diet. Others showed a partial response. Like others we have found that foods containing synthetic colouring material such as tartrazine, preservatives such as butylated hydroxy toluene and butylated hydroxy anisole (BHT & BHA) and foods containing natural salicylates are the main offenders.

2. Also like others we have found that many more boys than girls are affected. Of 214 children – 161 were boys. Males are known to have a higher requirement of Essential Fatty Acids than females.

3. A range of minor and sometimes major health problems repeatedly recurred in about four-fifths of our children. They included infantile colic, eczema, asthma, rhinitis, and repeated chest and ear infections.

4. We took hair samples from 31 boys and 15 girls and had them analysed by Dr P.J. Barlow of the Department of Environmental Health, University of Aston, Birmingham. 24 of 31 boys and 7 of 15 girls had zinc values below the normal range. Zinc is an important factor in the metabolism of Essential Fatty Acids.

5. About four-fifths of our children were **consistently thirsty**. This was particularly striking in families which contained normal children as well as a hyperactive one.

6. Some of our children who had not responded or had responded only partially to the Feingold diet did respond to a regime which eliminated **all milk and wheat products**.

7. There was a striking preponderance of fair- and ginger-haired children in the Survey Group.

8. SALICYLATES are known to block the formation of substances called PROSTAGLANDINS (PGs) and it was suggested that we should show our findings to a research scientist in Canada who has done work on PGs. He pointed out that many of our observations were consistent with the idea that HYPERACTIVE children might be deficient in PGs, notably PGE1 which is formed from the ESSENTIAL FATTY ACID dihomo-gamma-linolenic acid (DGLA). PGEI is extremely important for the control of the immune system, behaviour, the kidneys and thirst.

The Biochemical Steps in the Formation of PROSTAGLANDIN E1

CIS – LINOLEIC ACID (only from food intake)

Enzyme delta-6-desaturase needed for this first step (ZINC needed)

May be lacking in H.A. children

Blocked by trans – fatty acids, saturated fats, cholesterol, deficiencies of ZINC, INSULIN, MAGNESIUM, PYRIDOXINE (Vit. B_6 excess of alcohol, ageing, onocogenic viruses, chemical carcinogens, ionizing radiation)

1st STEP

DGLA STORE   gamma – linolenic acid   Pyridoxine possibly needed Vit. B_6

Zinc needed

2nd STEP

<u>Blocking agents</u>   di-homo gamma-linolenic acid   Ascorbic acid (Vit. C) niacin (Vit. B_3) needed

Salicylates
Tartrazine/Ponceau 4 R
(food dyes)
*Opioids of wheat and milk

3rd STEP

PROSTAGLANDIN E1

CONTROLS

IMMUNE SYSTEM	ASTHMA	BEHAVIOUR	KIDNEYS/THIRST

*Opioids are produced in the gut as a result of the digestion of wheat and milk

HACSG GENERAL INFORMATION SHEET

Almost ALL the babies and children the Hyperactive Children Support Group have had documented information on have responded well to the elimination of *additives*, especially *artificial colourings*, *preservatives* and *flavourings*.

Many of these children have come from families who have symptoms such as hayfever, eczema, asthma – especially migraine in mothers. Sometimes hayfever/migraine in fathers produces HA girls.

If the family has a background of 'atopy', it is possible that the child may have *intolerance* to some basic food(s) – the most likely one is cow's milk and products.

SOME EARLY SIGNS AND SYMPTOMS
1. Overactive in utero
2. Difficult birth
3. Atopic family (see above)
4. Colic
5. Diarrhoea
6. Ear problems
7. Wheezy chest
8. Catarrh
9. Migraine, eczema, asthma or hayfever in family or child.

Children from 'atopic' families who may suffer any of these problems might be intolerant – most likely foods are COW'S MILK or GLUTEN GRAINS.

Too many courses of antibiotics may interfere with metabolism of nutrients – cause malabsorption and upset the immune system further.

10. Reject mothering/cuddling/affection – maybe a 'miserable' baby
11. Very ticklish
12. Excessive thirst
13. Excessive dribbling/sweating/head sweats
14. Extra sensitive to noise (like Hoover/washing machine/loud noises)
15. Does not feel pain
16. Not aware of danger
17. Poor appetite, or gross appetite

18. Left-handed or ambidextrous
19. Head-banging (could be severe headaches)
20. Cot-rocking

Clinic vitamin drops and fluoride drops and tablets contain synthetic chemical additives and these can be very *un*helpful for babies and young children.

Many medicines contain colourings, flavourings and preservatives – all of which can cause severe reactions in these children. We must insist that additive-free medicine is made available.

Tap water in some areas can also cause severe problems (high nitrates/chlorine/lead/organophosphate pesticides/ over-high copper). For further information contact HACSG (see page 110 for address).

REPORTS ON EVENING PRIMROSE OIL, CO-FACTORS AND ZINC

REMARKS FROM HACSG PARENTS' REPORTS ON CHILDREN'S RESPONSE TO SUPPLEMENTS OF EVENING PRIMROSE OIL AND CO-FACTORS (ZINC, VITAMINS B AND C/MAGNESIUM)

- **Boy aged 2 years** 'Goes to bed easily at night on the first attempt and does not wake often in the night. We now have many uninterrupted nights. No nappy rash ... and seems much happier in himself.'
- **Boy aged 3 years** 'After 1–2 months was able to eat a less restricted diet without having any noticeable effects. Eczema and asthma somewhat better. My husband and I are thrilled with what the diet has achieved and that the world is at last able to see the lovable good child which we knew was always hiding in him. Results of infractions of the diet are not now so noticeable.'
- **Boy aged 4 years** 'Response almost immediate (3 days) improvements sustained. When zinc taken out, symptoms reappeared ... when zinc reintroduced, symptoms reduced again.'

- **Boy aged 4 years** 'Improvements seen after 1 week with evening primrose oil. After 2 weeks in general (including diet) improved speech, concentration, cooperation and understanding. Thirst back to normal.'
- **Boy aged 5 years** 'Hyperactivity lessened, allergies improved. Initially took 3–4 days to show response and overall improvement was marked.'
- **Boy aged 7 years** [*has Gilles de Tourett's Syndrome*] 'his tics have virtually disappeared since being on these supplements. This was noticeable in the first week. Concentration definitely improved.'
- **Boy aged 7 years** 'General behaviour better. Less tearful and irritable. Patch of eczema he had had for approx 1 year has almost gone completely.'
- **Boy aged 8 years** 'Eight-year-old catarrh problem had disappeared; constant thirst is normal now; easier to handle; less tantrums; better appetite. Diarrhoea and vomiting stopped; more colour in cheeks. School work improved on higher dose. Teacher said that there had been a big improvement in school work and behaviour getting good marks now.'
- **Boy aged 10 years** 'Improvement in both eczema and asthma (now off *Intal*) school reports increase in concentration. Less frustrated.'

Please contact the HACSG before giving Evening Primrose Oil to children under two years of age and to children/adults with epilepsy.

RECOMMENDED READING

Julian Barnard, *Bach Flower Remedies* (available from Holland & Barrett)

Dr Jonathan Brostoff and Linda Gamlin, *Food Allergy and Intolerance* (Bloomsbury)

H Cherry-Hills, *Good Food, Milk/Gluten Free* (Roberts Publications)

Dr William G Crook, *The Yeast Connection* (Professional Books)

Dr William Crook's Professional Booklets (available from HACSG, 71 Whyke Lane, Chichester, West Sussex PO19 2LD) include:
1. *Yeasts and their effect on your health*
2. *Allergy and your children*
3. *Hypoglycemia (low blood sugar)*

Dr William G Crook and Laura Stevens, *Solving the Puzzle of Your Hard to Raise Child* (Random House)

Adelle Davis, *Let's Eat Right to Keep Fit* (Allen and Unwin)

—, *Let's Get Well* (Allen and Unwin)

—, *Let's Have Healthy Children* (Allen and Unwin)

—, *Let's Stay Healthy: A guide to lifelong nutrition* (Allen and Unwin)

Robert Eagle, *Eating and Allergy* (Thorsons)

Dr Ben Feingold, *Why Your Child Is Hyperactive* (Random House)

Judy Graham and Dr M Odent, *The 'Z' Factor: How zinc is vital to your health* (Thorsons)

Dr Ellen Grant, *The Bitter Pill: How safe is the 'perfect contraceptive'?* (Corgi Books)

M Hannsen, *NEW 'E' for Additives* (Thorsons)

Professor Martin Herbert, *Behavioural Treatment of Children with Problems: A practical manual* (Academic Press)

Dr R MacKarness, *Chemical Victims* (Pan)

—, *Not All in the Mind* (Pan)

Dr Peter Mansfield and Dr Jean Monro, *Chemical Children: How to protect your family from harm* (Century Paperbacks)

Dr C Pfeiffer, *Zinc and Other Micro Nutrients* (Keats)

Miriam Polunin, *Minerals, What They Are and Why We Need Them* (Thorsons)

Doris J Rapp, MD, *Allergies and the HA Child* (Simon & Schuster)

Dr V Rippere, *The Allergy Problem* (Thorsons)

Dulcie Roberts and Janet Ash, *Hyperactive Child Cookbook* (available from HACSG, see above for address)

Dr Lendon H Smith, *Improving Your Child's Behaviour Chemistry* (Simon & Schuster)

Dr A Stewart and Dr S Davies, *Nutritional Medicine* (Pan)

Dr Roger J Williams, *Nutrition Against Disease* (Bantam)

Miriam Wood, *Living with a Hyperactive Child* (Souvenir Press)

Margaret and Arthur Wynn, *Prevention of Handicap and the Health of Women* (Routledge and Kegan Paul)

Many useful books are available from the following book-shops:

Merton Books
PO Box 279
Twickenham
Middlesex TW1 4XQ
A very wide range of books on nutrition, allergies, hyper-activity and many other related subjects. Please write for up-to-date book list.

Wholefood Books
24 Paddington Street
London W1
A very good stock of books on nutrition, allergy, hyper-activity, etc. Please write for an up-to-date price list of books available.

USEFUL ADDRESSES

Please send an SAE when contacting these Societies

The Hyperactive Children's Support Group
Sally Bunday
71 Whyke Lane
Chichester
West Sussex PO19 2LD

ALLERGY AND ASTHMA

Action Against Allergy
Greyhound House
23/24 George Street
Richmond
Surrey TW9 1JY

Allergy Care
Pollards Yard
Wood Street
Taunton
Somerset TA1 1UP
Tel. 01823 325 023 (enquiries)
(allergy testing)

Larkhall Green Farm
225 Putney Bridge Road
London SW15 2PY
Tel. 0181 874 1130
(facilities for allergy testing)

National Association for Research into Allergies
PO Box 45
Hinckley
Leicester LE10 1JY

National Asthma Campaign
Providence House
Providence Place
London N1 0NT
Tel. 0171 226 2260

AUTISM

Allergy Induced Autism
3 Palmera Avenue
Calcot
Reading
Berkshire RG3 7DZ

The International Autistic Research Organisation
49 Orchard Avenue
Shirley
Croydon CR0 7NE
Tel. 0171 777 0095

CHILD HEALTH, NUTRITION AND WELFARE

Foresight (Association for Preconceptual Care)
Mrs P Barnes
28 The Paddock
Godalming
Surrey GU7 1XD
Tel. 01483 427 839

Friends of the Earth
26–28 Underwood Street
London N1 7JQ
Tel. 0171 490 1555
(free publication list)

Nutrition Associates
Galtres House
Lysander Close
York YO3 8XB

The Organic Food Service
Ashe
Churston Ferrers
Brixham
Devon
(will provide addresses of local suppliers of organically-grown food)

The Soil Association
86 Colston Street
Bristol BS1 5BB
Tel. 01272 290 661
(has lists of organic suppliers)

CHILDREN WITH DISABILITIES

Association for Speech Impaired Children (AFASIC)
347 Central Markets
Smithfield
London EC1A 9NH
Tel: 0171 236 3632/6487

The British Institute for Brain Injured Children
Knowle Hall
Knowle
Bridgwater
Somerset TA7 8PJ

In-Touch
Anne Worthington
10 Norman Road
Sale
Cheshire M33 3DF
(scheme for parents of children with disabilities)

MENCAP
123 Golden Lane
London EC14 0RT

Network '81
The Voluntary Resource Centre
Latton Bush Centre
Southern Way
Harlow
Essex CM18
*(national network of parents and children with special
educational needs)*

The Research Trust for Metabolic Diseases in Children
53 Beam Street
Nantwich
Cheshire CW5 5NF
Tel. 01270 629 782

DYSLEXIA

British Dyslexia Association
98 London Road
Reading
Berkshire RG1 5AU
Helpline 0118 966 8271

Dyslexia Institute
133 Gresham Road
Staines
Middlesex TW18 2AJ

Hornsby Dyslexia Centre
71 Wandsworth Common
Westside
London SW18 2ED
Tel. 0181 871 2691

Helen Arkell Dyslexia Centre
Tel. 01251 254 446

A.C.E. (Advisory Centre for Education)
Unit 1B Aberdeen Studios
22–24 Highbury Grove
London N5 2EA
Tel. 0171 354 8321 (Mon–Fri 2–5 pm)

DYSLEXIA/DYSPRAXIA

New Research on Essential Fatty Acids:
Dr Jackie Stordy
Tel. 01483 402 665
or c/o Efamol Nutrition
Wyvern House
Wyvern Park
Portsmouth Road
Peasmarsh
Guildford GU3 1NA

ECZEMA

National Eczema Society
4 Tavistock Place
London WC1H 9RA
Tel. 0171 388 4097

HOMOEOPATHY

Ainsworths Homeopathic Pharmacy
38 New Cavendish Street
London W1M 7LH
Tel. 0171 935 5330 (3 lines)

British Homeopathic Association
27a Devonshire Street
London W1N 1RJ
Tel. 0171 935 2163

A. Nelson & Co Ltd
5 Endeavour Way
Wimbledon
London SW19 9UH

OSTEOPATHY

The General Council and Register of Osteopaths
56 London Street
Reading
Berkshire RG1 4SQ
Tel. 0118 957 6585
(to end of 1997 only)

Osteopathic Centre for Children
Administrative Centre
Honeysuckle Cottage
Inkpen Lane, Forest Row
East Sussex RH18 5BQ
Tel. 01342 824 466
(has a London clinic: tel: 0171 495 1231. Payment by small donation)

SUPPLIERS OF SUPPLEMENTS
AND VITAMINS

BioCare Ltd
'Lakeside'
180 Lifford Lane
Kings Norton
Birmingham B30 4NT

Bio-Health Ltd
Culpeper Close
Medway City Estate
Rochester
Kent ME2 4HU
Tel. 01634 290 115

Evening Primrose Oil
Send SAE and 65p in stamps to the Hyperactive
Children's Support Group (address above) for information
and their 'Parents Notes and Dosage' range.

G & G Vitamin Centre
51 Railway Approach
East Grinstead
West Sussex RH19 1BT

Larkhall Green Farm
(see above for address)

Nature's Best
FREEPOST
PO Box 1
Tunbridge Wells TW1 1XQ

Mrs P Aschwanden
'Vitamin Service'
Dellrose Cottage
Littlewick Road
Knaphill
Woking
Surrey GU21 2JU
Tel. 01483 488 845

GOVERNMENT DEPARTMENTS

Department for Education and Employment
Sanctuary Buildings
Great Smith Street
Westminster
London SW1P 3BT

Department of Health (general enquiries)
Richmond House
79 Whitehall
London SW1A 2NS

Ministry of Agriculture, Fisheries and Food (MAFF)
3 Whitehall Place
London SW1A 2HH